Management of Labor

Physician Judgment and Patient Care

Management of Labor

Physician Judgment and Patient Care

Mortimer G. Rosen

Willard C. Rappleye Professor of Obstetrics and Gynecology
Chairman of the Department
College of Physicians and Surgeons of Columbia University
Director of Obstetrics and Gynecology
Sloane Hospital for Women
Columbia-Presbyterian Medical Center
New York, New York

Elsevier
New York • Amsterdam • London

No responsibility is assumed by the Publisher for any injury and/or damage to persons or property as a matter of products liability, negligence, or otherwise, or from any use or operation of any methods, products, instructions, or ideas contained in the material herein. No suggested test or procedure should be carried out unless, in the reader's judgment, its risk is justified. Because of rapid advances in the medical sciences, we recommend that the independent verification of diagnoses and drug dosages should be made. Discussions, views, and recommendations as to medical procedures, choice of drugs, and drug dosages are the responsibility of the authors.

Elsevier Science Publishing Co., Inc.
655 Avenue of the Americas, New York, New York 10010

Sole distributors outside the United States and Canada:

Elsevier Science Publishers B.V.
P.O. Box 211, 1000 AE Amsterdam, The Netherlands

This book has been printed on acid-free paper.

Library of Congress Cataloging-in-Publication Data

Rosen, Mortimer G.
Management of labor : physician judgment and patient care / Mortimer G. Rosen.
p. cm.
ISBN 0-444-01528-0 (alk. paper)
1. Labor (Obstetrics) 2. Labor, Complicated. 3. Medical care—Decision making. 4. Judgment. I. Title.
[DNLM: 1. Delivery. 2. Judgment. 3. Labor. WQ 300 R813m]
RG651.R67 1990
618.4—dc20
DNLM/DLC
for Library of Congress 89-71491
CIP

Current printing (last digit):

10 9 8 7 6 5 4 3 2 1

Manufactured in the United States of America

This book is dedicated to
the clinician who applies the art of obstetrics
to the care of two patients during labor,
and who promises the best judgment,
but cannot guarantee a perfect outcome.

Contents

Preface *ix*
Acknowledgments *xi*

Chapter **1**
Crisis in the Labor Room: Understanding Morbidity and Mortality in the Management of Labor 1

Chapter **2**
Infant Brain Damage: Linkage with Labor 6

Chapter **3**
A Guide to Care in Labor 19

Chapter **4**
The Clinical Examination 37

Chapter **5**
The Latent Phase of Labor 47

Chapter **6**
The Treatment of Latent Phase Labor Abnormalities 62

Chapter **7**
The Active Phase and the Second Stage of Labor 86

Chapter **8**
The Second Stage of Labor 105

Chapter **9**
The Management of Active Phase and Second Stage Labor Abnormalities 123

Chapter **10**
Dystocia: The Pathology of Labor 138

Chapter **11**
Obstetrical Forceps: The Historical Background and the Debate 153

Chapter **12**
Forceps: Practical Considerations 158

Chapter **13**
Breech Presentation: The Controversy 172

Chapter **14**
Breech Presentation: The Delivery 180

Chapter **15**
In Summary: A Philosophy of Labor Management 194

Index *197*

Preface

Medical care is often not limited to a single treatment. At the bedside, several options for patient care may be present. The selection of the best treatment option, in large part, involves judgment. The use of good judgment, to the best of his or her ability, is explicit in the physician's oath. However, judgment is fallible. Therefore, a perfect outcome is always a goal to be sought, but not always an outcome which can be reached.

There are several purposes in this clinical text, the first of which is to present standard definitions or a dictionary of terms so that a common language may be used with universal understanding. Then, options for clinical choices that describe a philosophy for labor management will be presented. Labor management always involves several clinical choices.

If all obstetricians were to use the same definitions to describe the events of labor, this would lead to better understanding of all obstetrical practices. The standard set of definitions would simplify outcome comparisons between the several choices in medical practice. In turn, the ability to compare results would lead to more reasoned methods for improved clinical care.

In this text, definitions will be presented so that all clinicians will speak the same language. For instance, the word "dystocia" has little meaning. Chapter 9 is dedicated to reviewing the many uses of this word and the resulting confusion this term causes. Replace "dystocia" with the phrase "arrest in active phase labor" that can be defined, understood, measured and conveys more meaning.

In presenting protocols for patient care in this text, when complete information is lacking, it will be noted. For example, except in the most indirect manner, the electronic fetal heart monitor does not evaluate the brain and cannot provide direct information about fetal brain damage. Monitoring devices display fetal heart rate data and maternal uterine contraction activity that relate to fetal risk and potential for acidosis. The link to damage occurring in the brain at the time of monitoring cannot be made.

When more than one clinical choice is present, the several choices will be described. It is apparent that clinical care often involves several choices. Therefore, absolutes or rules are often limiting. Absolutes omit the art of judgment, and in individual patient care situations absolute rules rarely are appropriate. Guidelines suggest flexibility and allow more latitude.

If obstetricians cannot maintain the art of patient care, then the art may soon disappear. Obstetrical care will be diminished by the loss of decision choices and judgment. It is important that attention be paid to certain realities in this specialty. The vaginal birth route is not the alternative birth route. The correct cesarean birth rate is not known. The key for the clinician is choice followed by a judgment that is based on what is known.

This book is not written to replace standard texts, nor is it meant to serve as an encyclopedia of information. Rather, it represents a philosophy of and guidelines to patient care.

Acknowledgments

The author would like to express his appreciation to the many persons who made this book possible. First, Dr. David Peisner, whose meticulous review of the Friedman protocols in the Cleveland Metropolitan General Hospital data set helped confirm their accuracy and allowed a philosophy of pregnancy care to be based on both data and reason. Second, there were other members of the faculty at the Cleveland Metropolitan General Hospital who both by their care for the data systems and their practice of obstetrics allowed us to practice what we preached. These include Dr. Lawrence Chik, Dr. Roger Hertz, Dr. Robert Sokol, Dr. Leroy Dierker, Dr. Ilan Timor, Dr. Sydney Bottoms, and Mr. Victor Hirsh.

The manuscript preparation and indefatigable support of Ms. Reba Nosoff is gratefully acknowledged.

Finally, without the continuing encouragement of my wife, Dr. Lynn Rosen, who kept telling me to "write it as you speak it," this book would not have been completed.

Chapter 1

Crisis in the Labor Room

Understanding Morbidity and Mortality in the Management of Labor

OVERVIEW

The Crisis

Today there is much confusion in obstetrical practice concerning the effect of medical interventions during labor on infant outcome. This is illustrated by the high cesarean birthrates in order to lower infant mortality, and by the continuing increase in cesarean birthrates of more than 1.5% each year.[1]

In 1984, the estimated total cesarean birthrate was about 21.2%.[2] In 1987, the estimated cesarean rate rose to 25%. In order to justify this operative intervention, maternal and perinatal morbidity and mortality should document continuing improvement in maternal and fetal outcomes corresponding with the rising cesarean birthrate.

Although remarkable decreases in death and damage to mother and fetus have taken place during the past 30 years, the maternal and fetal improvement in outcome is not directly related to the cesarean birthrate. Most cesareans are performed in healthy women at term. Maternal morbidity and mortality studies depict this quite well. The quality of obstetrical care far transcends the cesarean birth. It is this type of assumed cause and effect relationship, as well as the external forces of patient and society, which confronts the physician and has helped to create confusion in clinical practice. The crisis is that continuing intervention is not leading to continuing improvement in maternal and fetal outcome.

OBJECTIVES

At the conclusion of this chapter, the clinician should understand the relationships between:

1. Cesarean delivery and patient outcome
2. Maternal risk and obstetrical intervention
3. Fetal risk and obstetrical intervention
4. Patients' expectations and their influences on care
5. Fear of litigation and its influence on obstetrical intervention

MATERNAL MORTALITY RATES

For many years maternal mortality conferences were a part of every hospital's teaching program. They set the standards for clinicians seeking better understanding and new methods for avoiding maternal deaths. In the 20th century maternal mortality has continued to decrease. In 1935 maternal mortality rates were 582 per 100,000 live births; they fell to 8.9 per 100,000 live births by 1982. During 1982 there were more than 5.6 million births with an estimated 330 maternal deaths.[3]

Deaths had become so infrequent that maternal mortality conferences fell into disuse. Conferences related to maternal and fetal medical complications during pregnancy replaced mortality concerns.

As an example of this changing focus of obstetrics, during 1982 in the city of Philadelphia one citywide maternal mortality conference was held, and that conference was held only at the insistence of an interested physician who had recently moved to Philadelphia (Personal Communication, Dr. Jan Schneider, MD, Philadelphia, 1985). No citywide maternal mortality conference was held in the next several years. Today, although the classic etiologies for maternal deaths—hemorrhage, infection, and toxemia—are still present and important, they are being challenged by new maternal risk factors such as obstetrical complications involving cesarean surgery and, increasingly, anesthetic risk.[3]

MATERNAL MORTALITY DUE TO CESAREAN

Despite the fact that one Boston hospital could record more than 10,000 cesarean births without an operative-related maternal death, any use of anesthesia, no matter how expertly given, is less safe than no use of anesthesia.[4] In addition, although anesthetic care is generally at a high level of safety, its availability varies both with hospital size and number of obstetrical deliveries.

Untoward consequences of maternal morbidity following cesarean include infection, estimated to be between 20% and 40%, which exceeds the rate for maternal infections following spontaneous births.[5] In today's rapidly changing epidemiology of infection, the introduction of AIDS adds new risk factors. It is not unusual for a patient to tell the obstetrician that she fears infection by blood transfusion, which is an increased risk following cesarean surgery. The average blood loss following cesarean birth may exceed 1000 cc and is two to three times higher than blood loss following spontaneous vaginal birth.[3]

Review of available data documents maternal mortality following emergency cesarean as being 40.9 per 100,000 cesarean deliveries, four times the rate of maternal mortality following spontaneous birth. Even elective cesarean carries with it a twofold increase in maternal deaths.[6] Thus, while the cesarean is an extremely low-risk procedure, it is associated with increased maternal morbidity and mortality.

The maternal data may be summarized by noting that actual surgical risks for maternal death are extremely low, and have been remarkably improved through better understanding of surgical technique, anesthetic use, blood transfusion, and treatment of infection. Yet the many inherent forms of morbidity in this procedure do not support the statement made that there is little difference in maternal risk between vaginal birth and cesarean birth.

FETAL RISK REPLACES MATERNAL RISK

Fetal care often replaces maternal care as our primary focus in today's obstetrics. As noted, because maternal risk from the cesarean is small, the clinical choice for cesarean is far easier and allows for greater freedom of choice when considering the more complicated birth events such as the breech birth, the delivery of twins, and the use of obstetrical midforceps. The driving force behind most clinical decisions during labor today is a concern for the quality of life for the fetus. Avoidance of intrapartum fetal brain damage, which may appear later in infancy as cerebral palsy, is a high priority. Because of its influence on patient care, the specific issue of infant brain damage is addressed in Chapter 2. The prevalence of cerebral palsy from all causes today is estimated to be between one and three affected children per 1000 children at 7 to 20 years of age; one half of those following premature birth.[7]

Perinatal mortality has continued to decrease and this change suggests improvement in fetal and neonatal therapy. Less clear is what specific factors contribute most to the improved infant outcomes. For example, in New York State from 1968 to 1977, perinatal mortality rates fell and cesarean birthrates increased almost in parallel. This could suggest a related effect of the rising cesarean birthrate on infant outcome. During the second half of the 1968 to 1977 time period, the cesarean birthrate continued to increase, but the perinatal mortality rates decreased much more slowly.[6] This obviously makes the idea of a close relationship between more cesareans and improved infant outcome a tenuous concept.

As we approach the goal of lowered risk and morbidity, the size of the high-risk target population becomes smaller; therefore, the identification of the at-risk fetus becomes more difficult. Today a large percentage of the fetal-risk population lies in the under 1500 g low-birth-weight group. This low-birth-weight group probably contributes to more than 75% of perinatal mortality, although the low-birth-weight population (less than 2500 g) accounts for less than 5% to 12% of all births.[8] Operative intervention as the major method for improving infant outcome would not remove all or even most causes of brain damage or infant morbidity in this low-birth-weight population. The question of how many cesareans are justified to approach our goals of diminished maternal and perinatal morbidity is not clear.

PATIENTS' EXPECTATIONS OF A PERFECT OUTCOME AND MALPRACTICE ACCUSATIONS

Complicating the treatment choices during labor is the patients' expectation of a perfect outcome. Anything less than a healthy infant raises the question of why did the morbidity occur? The clinicians' judgment and medical decisions are complicated by the fear of malpractice accusations and the associated emotional and financial risks.

There are few practicing obstetricians who have not been queried or deposed by a plaintiff's attorney. All obstetricians know of associates who have been sued in poor outcome situations. The physician's personal distress may be so profound that even when the clinician believed that the patient care was correct, by the end of a deposition or trial, or after many months of reevaluation, both in public and in private, personal doubts may have been created. For that physician the safer choice the "next time" may be an attempt to reach a "lower risk" personal situation sooner. In these cases, the decision is usually made for a cesarean. Almost all published reports indicate cesarean birthrates are higher in private practice environments than among the non-private practice population despite the fact that the latter population is at higher medical risk.

To the obstetrician practicing in this arena, four rules for patient care and malpractice risk are offered.

1. If you practice good obstetrics and maternal and infant outcome is good, you will not be sued.
2. If you practice poor obstetrics (not recommended) and maternal and fetal outcome is good, you will not be sued.
3. If you practice good obstetrics and either maternal or fetal outcome is poor, you will be sued.
4. If you practice poor obstetrics and either maternal or fetal outcome is poor, you will be sued.

Therefore, if you are to be sued on the basis of clinical *outcome*, not on the basis of clinical *care*, why not practice good obstetrics?

SUMMARY

1. Change of medical practice in obstetrics must be justified by improved outcome for mother and fetus.
2. Morbidity and mortality rates for the neonate and the mother have improved markedly during the 20th century. The rise in cesarean births during the past 15 years cannot easily be linked with the decrease in morbidity.
3. The cesarean, a relatively safe procedure, carries increased risk for the mother in present and future pregnancies.
4. The cesarean is a safe birth route for the fetus of the present pregnancy, but carries increased risk for the fetus of a future pregnancy.

REFERENCES

1. Shiono PH, Fielden JG, McNellis D, et al: Recent trends in cesarean birth and trial of labor rates in the U.S. JAMA 1987;257:494–497.
2. Shiono PH, McNellis DM, Rhoads GG: Reasons for the rising cesarean delivery rates: 1978–1984. Obstet Gynecol 1987;69:696–700.
3. Pritchard JA, MacDonald PC, Grant N: Williams Obstetrics, ed 17. Norwalk, CT, Appleton-Century-Crofts, 1985, pp 3, 193, 356.
4. Frigoletto FD Jr, Ryan KJ, Phillipe M: Maternal mortality rate associated with cesarean section: an appraisal. Am J Obstet Gynecol 1980;136:969–970.
5. Merril BS, Gibbs CE: Planned vaginal delivery following cesarean section. Obstet Gynecol 1978;52:50–52.
6. Cesarean Childbirth, publication 82-2067. Bethesda, MD, National Institutes of Health, October, 1981, pp 159–239, 255–279.
7. Freeman, J: Prenatal and perinatal factors associated with brain disorders, publication 85-1149. Bethesda, MD, National Institutes of Health, April 1985, p 430.
8. Holbrook RH Jr, Creasy RK. Prevention of preterm delivery, Postgrad Med 1984;75:177–185.

Chapter 2

Infant Brain Damage

Linkage with Labor

OVERVIEW

In the Introduction it was noted that one of the forces modulating the changing clinical care of women during labor was the concern, of both physician and patient, with the later appearance of infant brain damage. This infant pathology is often defined in three major categories: mental retardation, epilepsy, and cerebral palsy. Although there are other forms of brain dysfunction, because of lack of data it is not possible to attribute etiologies in other brain functions, such as behavioral problems or learning disorders, to the intrapartal period.

These three major neurologic categories—cerebral palsy, epilepsy, and mental retardation—will be discussed as distinct and separate entities. Cerebral palsy is a nonprogressive motor dysfunction which may include mental retardation and convulsions. It is an illness which is different from pure epilepsy or pure mental retardation.

In this chapter the pathophysiology of brain injury will be reviewed and linked, when possible, to the potential risk for damage during labor. Attention will also be directed to the association with brain damage of fetal distress, fetal acidosis, and Apgar scores. For a more complete review of prenatal and perinatal events as they relate to brain damage, the reader is referred to a review entitled *Prenatal and Perinatal Factors Associated with Brain Disorders* published in 1985 by the National Institute of Health[1] and summarized in a review article.[2]

OBJECTIVES

At the conclusion of this chapter, the clinician should understand the following:

1. Pathologic findings associated with infant brain damage
2. Brain damage syndromes associated with obstetrical care
3. The relationships between brain damage and
   a. Intrapartal asphyxia
   b. Apgar scores
   c. Birth route
   d. Fetal distress

PATHOPHYSIOLOGY OF ASPHYXIAL BRAIN DAMAGE

Reasons for Confusion

The causes for the death of brain cells in the fetal and neonatal brain are still unclear. As they relate to obstetrical interventions during labor, gross neurologic injuries may be divided into those associated with asphyxia and, less frequently, those injuries associated with direct fetal trauma.

Other clinical problems such as infection or genetic defects are not included in this review. The term "asphyxia" is identified with poorly understood modifiers such as acute or chronic asphyxia, or perinatal, neonatal, or intrapartal asphyxia. These words may identify a length of time or a period of life, but they are vague. For example, perinatal asphyxia extends from 28 weeks of fetal life to 28 days of neonatal life. This term adds little information as to when an injury to the brain may have developed. It does not give us a day of injury or a cause for the damage. It merely describes a long period of time during which an event may have occurred.

The words "anoxia" or "asphyxia" may be well-defined in textbooks, but are not used with precision in the clinical arena. Certainly there is risk for brain damage with asphyxia or anoxia. How much asphyxia must be present before brain damage occurs, or what other factors may increase the fetal and neonatal risk for actual damage, are not well understood. Unfortunately, the use of these terms implies that damage will occur and that is usually an incorrect assumption.

EXAMPLE OF FETAL SUPPLY RISK CONFOUNDED BY PREMATURITY AND LABOR

Long-standing, poor placental supply in a chronic hypertensive mother was associated with a severely growth-retarded fetus at labor onset at 32 weeks of gestation. Onset of labor monitoring revealed late fetal heart rate decelerations.

Comment

The preexisting supply problem may be a greater risk for morbidity than the superimposed acute fetal supply problem during labor documented by the late decelerations. There is no clinical information separating the acute from the chronic events. In addition, the same degree of uteroplacental insufficiency in the term fetus may result in different effects from those that occur in the very low-birth-weight fetus, as it did in this example. The associated risks of anoxia, maturity, and labor cannot easily be assessed.

The term "may" is used cautiously. Immaturity has always been spoken of as a time period of greater resistance to cell death when compared with older organisms. However, problems such as intracerebral hemorrhage occur more often at the lowest birth weights. In these examples, deprivation of fetal supply is inferred. What cannot be answered in the above example is whether the fetal brain was injured during the prenatal period when it was not growing well, during labor when the stress was acute, or during both time periods with one risk being added to a second risk.

EXAMPLE OF ABNORMAL LABOR CONFOUNDED BY ABNORMAL FETAL HEART RATE PATTERN

A term mother undergoes an arrest in the active phase of labor followed by a series of deep variable decelerations as she enters the second stage of labor. Is that fetus more vulnerable to brain damage following a series of variable fetal heart rate decelerations than a fetus facing variable decelerations during a normal active phase labor?

Comment

These confounding variables raise obvious questions, but answers to those questions are not known. The two problems may be additive or they may add no increased risk, yet the obstetrician more often intervenes in the abnormal labor situation. The diagnosis of dystocia with fetal distress is a frequent one. Risk for neurologic damage in the presence of dystocia alone is quite low and is described more completely in Chapter 10.

NEUROPATHOLOGY OF ASPHYXIAL BRAIN DAMAGE

The early endpoints of the potentially morbid perinatal problems of asphyxia are seen by the clinician as intracranial bleeding and edema. The endpoints after the acute problem are visualized as nerve death, gross morphologic change, and altered neurologic function of the child. The evolution from early signs to later development and function cannot be predicted with great accuracy.

EXAMPLE OF EVOLUTION OF NEUROPATHOLOGIC EVENTS

In a term fetus a prolonged compression of the umbilical cord was associated with the birth of a severely depressed Apgar 2, 4, infant. Cerebral edema, subarachnoid, and intraventricular hemorrhage were later visualized on ultrasonographic studies during the first several days of life. Clinical signs of neurologic dysfunction were seen during the first 12 hours. Seizures occurred during the next several days. At the time of discharge the neonate appeared to be feeding well, and the seizures were controlled by medication. During the neonatal period, prediction of future development was not easily made, and the diagnosis was guarded at the time of discharge.

Comment

Unfortunately, because of the cell death in the baby's brain, the neonate which had been normocephalic at birth was microcephalic 1 year later. By that time the diagnosis was certain, and the child did have cognitive and motor pathology.

To describe this pathology, broad classifications, which include hemorrhage and edema, are used.[1,3] In the case of fetal and neonatal bleeding, there are three general categories of bleeding: subdural, subarachnoid, and intracerebral. For purposes of simplifying this discussion, the cephalhematoma, or extracranial bleed, which often occurs spontaneously or in association with trauma, rarely causes brain damage and will not be described.

Subdural Hemorrhage

The subdural bleed, or subdural hematoma, is a lesion which is relatively uncommon in today's obstetrics because of the trend to avoid traumatic labors. During the last 25 years, the practice of obstetrics has turned away from the use of the high or difficult midforceps, or the acceptance of excessively prolonged labors. Thus, this category, once prominent, is now uncommon.

In association with the subdural bleed there are lacerations of the larger veins of the dura mater. When the subdural hemorrhage occurs, it is seen in the term fetus more frequently than in the low-birth-weight fetus, and is often associated with physical trauma to the fetal head. The classic clinical picture associated with this pathology will occur in a patient who has had a difficult forceps application following a protraction or arrest in the active phase of labor, or following a delay in descent of the vertex. The hematoma, or bleed, may be associated with a skull fracture, but usually this is not present. The neonate often becomes depressed shortly after birth and as the neonate recovers from the trauma, it begins to display signs of abnormal neurologic function such as changes in muscle tone, irritability, and seizures. This subdural hemorrhage is frequently associated with severe infant developmental pathology such as cerebral palsy, with motor and cognitive dysfunction.

Subarachnoid Hemorrhage

This cerebral bleed is more frequently seen than the subdural hemorrhage. This hemorrhage may be isolated to the subarachnoid space, or it may be seen in association with intracerebral bleeding. Although on occasion the subarachnoid bleeding may be associated with trauma, usually it is found along with clinical signs of fetal distress which precipitated the intervention in the first place.

Most subarachnoid hemorrhages are diagnosed in the neonate and are associated with clinical fetal risk conditions such as acidosis or asphyxia. Perhaps three quarters of all subarachnoid hemorrhages will be seen in the lowest birth weight neonates with the remaining 25% being seen in term infants.[3] These bleeds may also be found unassociated with known risks of labor.

Usually the subarachnoid bleed relates to some form of fetal deprivation of supply. The term asphyxia is a more specific supply problem. These terms do not completely overlap. The term "deprivation of supply" includes not only cell respiratory problems, such as asphyxia, but all metabolic problems as well, including nutritional deprivation as seen in intrauterine growth retardation. Several confounding clinical events may be present and confuse the etiology of the subarachnoid hemorrhage.

EXAMPLE OF CONFOUNDING RISK FOR SUBARACHNOID HEMORRHAGE

Intrapartal fetal distress occurred in a growth-deprived 1753-g infant. During the neonatal period the infant had severe respiratory distress and neonatal asphyxia.

Comment

Which risks caused this infant's damage? The brain was already at risk because of the prenatal problem of growth retardation. This was confounded by preterm birth and intrapartal fetal distress. Later, the neonatal risks of respiratory distress and asphyxia occurred. Are these risks linked, cumulative, or independent? In individual cases, the answers to these questions are often unclear.

Subarachnoid bleeding usually occurs during the neonatal period, the time when most brain hemorrhage occurs. The confusion in the association of several risk factors makes it difficult to assign risk in other than a general manner.[4] All of these individual clinical risks are potentially harmful. All of these associations may increase the risk for pre-subarachnoid bleeding. First causes for these problems are not easily documented. Stated differently, the presence of intrapartal fetal distress seen during electronic monitoring may be a result of already present damage or a cause of the damage.

Intracerebral Hemorrhage

Although originally noted to take place around the cerebral ventricles and called periventricular leukoencephalomalacia, intracerebral bleeding also takes place away from the ventricles and within all areas of the brain.[5,6] Intracerebral bleeding is most frequently associated with prematurity. The lowest birth weight fetuses (<1500 g) have the highest incidence of periventricular and intracerebral bleeding.[6] We do not know how to avoid this injury. One clinical question, which at this writing is yet unanswered, is whether the physiologic problems of prematurity can be overcome by altering the fetal birth route. This raises the question of whether there is any birth weight below which the cesarean is the procedure of choice? Stated differently, is the physical pressure on the brain during vaginal birth an increased risk for intracerebral bleeding? Does asphyxia occur more often in low-birth-weight fetuses because of an intolerance to labor?

The answer to the pathophysiology of these intracerebral hemorrhages may lie in the maturity of fetal blood vessels.[3] The immature blood vessels in the developing brain of a low-birth-weight fetus or neonate are no more than several cells thick. When exposed to stress associated with asphyxia and acidosis, or pressure on the vertex, or both stresses, the intracerebral circulation changes and flow through the smaller blood vessels may stop as the blood pressure falls. Without blood flow, these thin-walled vessels may become damaged due to lack of supply. When circulation is restored, blood flows through these damaged vessels and intracerebral bleeding occurs.

This intracerebral hemorrhage is closely linked with fetal immaturity. It may also occur in association with neonatal events such as continuous positive airway pressure and neonatal respiratory distress.[6]

The suggestion that alteration of birth route—by using the cesarean and avoiding labor—will alter intracerebral bleeding has not been demonstrated.[7] Advocates for both birth-route choices still exist. A stronger argument may be made that the treatment of intracerebral hemorrhage should be the prevention of premature birth.

Grading Intracerebral Hemorrhage

Intracerebral bleeding has been divided into four categories:

Grade 1: Bleeding in the periventricular zone

Grade 2: Bleeding in the periventricular zone distorting the outline of the ventricles

Grade 3: Bleeding in the periventricular zone distorting the ventricles and with rupture

Grade 4: Bleeding in the periventricular zone, distorting the ventricles, rupturing into ventricles, and with associated bleeding into the brain substance

Infant neurologic evaluations document that signs of infant clinical brain damage will more often be found in association with grade 3 and 4 hemorrhages. In grades 1 and 2 bleeds, brain damage is less commonly found.[1]

Cerebral Edema

In the past, cerebral edema was less frequently identified by physical examination, fontanel tenseness, and increased spinal fluid pressure. Today, cerebral edema is more easily and more frequently found with the use of computerized tomography or ultrasonography. With these diagnostic techniques, much more information is available about the presence of cerebral edema. In the past, edema was often overlooked.

Cerebral edema occurs more frequently in the term infant than the preterm infant. It is usually associated with difficult labor or fetal distress. Although hemorrhage may also occur in term infants, as a general statement, bleeding is seen more frequently in the less mature fetus and edema more frequently with maturity.[3] Again, depending on the severity of the events which lead to the edema, there may be varying degrees of brain damage and risk for abnormal brain development. Intracerebral edema represents a reaction to an injury and may be associated with cell necrosis.

ASSOCIATION OF PATHOLOGY WITH FUNCTION

Brain Plasticity

In all attempts to correlate pathology with later malfunction, several confounding problems must be considered. In the first, called "plasticity of the brain," the brain may have sufficient reserve or new resources for compensating for the damage. This plasticity implies an ability of a new area of the brain to take over a function for the damaged area. Attempts to quantitate motor or cognitive effects of a potentially injurious event may be limited when the pathology is small and when an alternate area of the brain assumes or relearns the lost function. The question of how many cells must be damaged before brain damage can be recognized is unanswerable. Each organ has a great deal of reserve function. The expression of and the testing for intellectual, behavioral, or motor ability in the neonate or infant is limited. In the neonatal period there are no accepted useful clinical tests which, when given during the first few days of life, predict later intelligence or motor ability. A neonatal brain may be damaged and at risk for cerebral palsy because of damaging events. Many months or even years may pass before cerebral palsy is identified clinically.

Linkage of Specific Cerebral Pathology with Clinical Damage

As already noted, the presence of brain hemorrhage, or edema, is not always associated with neurologic damage. Why some infants adapt to the bleed and perform normally and yet, following the same clinical events other infants are damaged, is not clear. Even more confusing is the fact that "perinatal asphyxia," or "asphyxia neonatorum," has been identified as being the cause of many infant neurologic diseases extending from cerebral palsy through the learning disorders.[1]

Autopsy studies have found that the same intracerebral pathology does not always follow a single etiologic factor. Conversely, 28 different morphologic brain abnormalities have been attributed to the same clinical function or illness, asphyxia.[1] The problem may be diagrammed as follows:

Confusion in Understanding Infant Brain Damage

Same cerebral pathology is associated with many clinical forms of damage
Different clinical insults may result in a single area of brain damage
Different clinical events may result in perinatal asphyxia

The confusion in terms leaves the clinician perplexed when trying to prevent morbidity. Patient care techniques must be chosen, often without adequate etiologic information.

Neurologic Damage, Fetal Risk, and Fetal Maturity

Another factor obscuring the link between fetal risk and infant outcome is fetal maturity at the time risk occurs. The dynamic fetal condition, rapidly changing and evolving from a less mature organism to more mature organism in utero (or as a neonate), may in part explain the reasons for the confusion.

EXAMPLE OF SAME FETAL RISK OCCURRING AT DIFFERENT FETAL MATURITY STAGES, PRODUCING TWO DIFFERENT CLINICAL SYNDROMES CALLED CEREBRAL PALSY

The clinical findings of cerebral palsy that follows fetal brain injury which took place at 28 weeks of maturity are different from the clinical findings of cerebral palsy following brain injury which took place at 38 weeks of maturity. The infants have different motor and cognitive deficits when seen at 2 years of age. This indicates that different areas of the fetal brain have different levels of vulnerability to the same stimulus at different stages of life.

Comment

The low-birth-weight fetus may hemorrhage in response to prolonged umbilical cord compression. The term infant may display diffuse cortical edema in response to prolonged umbilical cord compression. The resulting injuries will occur in different parts of the brain. Both infants may express cerebral pathology. The same fetal asphyxial risk may lead to one clinical form of cerebral palsy in the low-birth-weight fetus, and a different clinical form of cerebral palsy in the term fetus. Thus, the same high-risk event at different times of human development leads to different forms of brain damage. The vulnerability of different areas of the brain varies with the stage of growth and development.

AVOIDING FETAL BRAIN DAMAGE

It is clear that brain injury may result from pathologic human development from the time of conception throughout the fetal period. In the majority of cases the clinician and the patient have the intuitive feeling that brain damage can be avoided by obstetrical interventions in and around labor. This concept is too narrow.

As noted in the recent report from the National Institutes of Health,[1] cytogenetic, biochemical, and teratogenic events, and many other intrauterine problems, such as deprivation of fetal supply and in utero fetal infections, are associated with the children already damaged or mentally retarded at the time of labor. The existing brain damage is unknown to the clinician who cannot test for in utero brain function.

EXAMPLE OF AN ALREADY DAMAGED FETUS NOT IMPROVED BY CESAREAN DELIVERY

If the breech presentation fetus is already damaged, that may be one of the reasons it moves differently in utero and assumes the breech position.

Comment

Most fetuses in breech presentations are neurologically normal. However, the incidence of preexisting fetal brain damage in this population is higher than that for the vertex presentation group (see Chapter 13). Therefore, all breech presentations are already at higher risk for morbidity than the vertex presentation of the same birth weight.

EXAMPLE OF AN ALREADY DAMAGED FETUS WHICH MAY EXHIBIT INTRAPARTAL FETAL DISTRESS

The growth retarded or postmature fetus with little metabolic reserve due to supply deprivation for the previous week will quickly show electronic monitoring signs of late decelerations when labor begins. Was brain damage present or did labor cause brain damage?

Comment

It is impossible to identify this damaged brain prior to birth. If this fetus is already damaged, it may react abnormally to labor and present with signs of acute fetal distress. The best clinical example is the fetal heart rate monitoring tracing in which there is absence of beat-to-beat variability when the fetal electronic monitor is first applied. In these cases there is confusion as to whether, in the presence of abnormal findings, the labor adds to the damage. Should a cesarean be performed immediately or should a trial of labor ensue? These are questions which cannot be answered.

INTRAPARTAL DAMAGE AND EARLY NEONATAL FUNCTION

In general, it is correct to expect that if the fetus was damaged intrapartally, the early neonatal period should be abnormal. Recent stress to the fetus of sufficient degree to cause brain damage is unlikely to leave the neonate with no signs of abnormality.[1] The converse of that statement is also true. If, during the neonatal period, observed function had been normal, the previously damaged but now recovered fetus reflects insults prior to labor.

Using a different model, if the fetal brain is damaged during the antepartum period, it may appear either normal or abnormal during the neonatal period. This depends on how well the fetus recovered from the in utero injury. If the injury took place antepartum, it may not be until much later in infancy until the clinical disability can be identified. Neonatal function often does not demonstrate clinical pathology.

RELATIONSHIP OF LABOR TO CEREBRAL PALSY, EPILEPSY, AND MENTAL RETARDATION

Cerebral Palsy

Cerebral palsy is a nonprogressive motor disorder, such as mental retardation, which may be associated with convulsions. In general, the infant with cerebral palsy is not mentally retarded.[8] Cerebral palsy may be associated with intrapartal events.

Estimates of the frequency of association between cerebral palsy and perinatal asphyxia varies from 25% to 51%.[1] About one half of the known causes of cerebral palsy occur following nonlabor events.[9] The majority of children who later show cerebral palsy have had normal Apgar scores.[1,10] A depressed Apgar score at 1 minute, but greater than 6 at 5 minutes is associated with no greater risk for cerebral palsy than a child with a normal Apgar score at 1 and 5 minutes.[10]

The misuse of the Apgar score occurs frequently. The score was never intended to predict brain damage. In a population of infants, a depressed Apgar score has statistical significance. For the individual neonate, the Apgar score is a poor predictor of development. The Apgar score should give direction for fetal treatment to the clinician, but it is not accurate for predicting neurologic function.

Epilepsy and Mental Retardation: Two Different Conditions Less Related to Intrapartal Risk

Epilepsy, a illness unassociated with other neuropathology, such as cerebral palsy, is rarely associated with the birth process.[1] The majority of the causes of epilepsy are unknown.[11] However, that is not the case with the severely damaged infant who also has convulsions in association with motor pathology; that is a diagnosis of cerebral palsy.

Mental retardation, defined as a purely cognitive deficit unassociated with epilepsy or cerebral palsy, is identified as being associated with intrapartal risk in less than 10% of the cases.[1] More often this pure defect reflects genetic or biochemical events which are not changed by intrapartal manipulations. An infant may have the same mental retardation cognitive effect in association with motor defects and convulsion. That syndrome is cerebral palsy.

SUMMARY

1. Pathologic findings associated with brain damage
   - A. Subdural hematoma
     1. Often associated with trauma
     2. Should rarely occur in intrapartal care
   - B. Subarachnoid hemorrhage
     1. Occurs more frequently in the low-birth-weight fetus (three times more than term fetus)
     2. May be associated with trauma or asphyxia
     3. May lead to brain damage
   - C. Intracerebral hemorrhage
     1. Occurs most frequently in the low-birth-weight fetus during neonatal period
     2. Associated with asphyxia and prematurity
     3. May lead to brain damage
   - D. Cerebral edema
     1. Seen more commonly in the term infant in the intrapartum period following stress
     2. May lead to brain damage
2. Brain damage syndromes linked with intrapartal care
   - A. Cerebral palsy
     1. 50% associated with perinatal risks
     2. 50% associated with low-birth-weight fetuses
     3. Significant overlap between categories 1 and 2
     4. Significant percentage follow normal gestations, labors without fetal risk, and have normal Apgar scores
   - B. Epilepsy as a pure disease is rarely associated with perinatal or intrapartal events
   - C. Mental retardation as a pure disease is rarely associated with perinatal or intrapartal events

3. Brain damage
   A. May be present in some fetuses before labor onset
   B. May be influenced by labor
   C. May occur in the neonatal period in association with prematurity

4. Apgar scores
   A. Do not correlate well with cerebral palsy
   B. Relate to intrapartal fetal distress

REFERENCES

1. Freeman J: Prenatal and perinatal factors associated with brain disorders, publication 85-1149. Bethesda, MD, National Institutes of Health, April, 1985.
2. Rosen MG, Hobel CJ: Prenatal and perinatal factors associated with brain disorders. Obstet Gynecol 1986; 68:416-421.
3. Pape KE, Wigglesworth SS: Hemorrhage, ischemia and the perinatal brain. London, Heinemann, 1979.
4. Rosen MG, Bilenker RM, Thompson K: An assessment of developmental time periods and risk for brain damage in fetus and infant. J Reprod Med 1986; 31:297-303.
5. Banker BQ, Larroche JC: Periventricular leukoencephalomalacia of infancy. A form of anoxic encephalopathy. Arch Neurol 1962; 7:386-410.
6. Pape KE, Armstrong DL, Fitzhardinge PM: Central nervous system pathology associated with mask ventilation in the very low birthweight infant: a new etiology of intracerebral hemorrhages. Pediatrics 1976; 58:473-483.
7. Westgren M, Paul R: Delivery of the low birth weight infant by cesarean section. Clin Obstet Gynecol 1985; 28:752-762.
8. Kiely M, Labin RA, Kiely JL: The descriptive epidemiology of cerebral palsy. Public Health Rev 1984; 12:79-101.
9. Hagberg G, Hagberg B, Chow I: The changing panorama of cerebral palsy in Sweden, 1954-1970. III. The importance of foetal deprivation of supply. Acta Paediatr Scand 1976; 65:403-408.
10. Nelson KB, Ellenberg JH: Apgar scores as predictors of cerebral palsy. Pediatrics 1981; 68:36-44.
11. Hauser WA, Kurland LT: Epidemiology of epilepsy in Rochester, Minn, 1935-1986. Epilepsia 1975; 16:1-66.

Chapter 3

A Guide to Care in Labor

OVERVIEW

Confusion in the use of terms such as perinatal and neonatal asphyxia, anoxia, and their relationships to the etiology of brain damage have been described. Terminology for labor and the definitions of labor diagnoses are used in this textbook as a dictionary of descriptive terms for patient care. If there are clinical definitions when normal clinical courses have been exceeded, it is easier to consider making intrapartal decisions. When you exceed usual points, you act. Actions must follow defined information, not just a feeling; for example, "the head won't fit." Cephalopelvic disproportion may be present but can only be speculated on even after the neonate has been delivered. In contrast, failure of the vertex to descend after full cervical dilatation is definable in terms of time.

In this text, Friedman's labor definitions have been used as they are derived from his original calculations performed at Presbyterian Hospital and Columbia University College of Physicians and Surgeons in New York.[1] In more recent studies of women during labor performed at Cleveland Metropolitan General Hospital by Dr. David Peisner together with the author, comparisons with Friedman's original observations were remarkably consistent.[2–4] In a few instances, such as in the latent phase of labor, practical clinical modifications will be introduced. However, throughout this text, the Friedman criteria are used as guidelines for documenting what is taking place. Clinical intervention, made in association with labor diagnosis, involves the use of good judgment performed at the bedside by the clinician. Too often the Friedman guidelines have been used as a reason for terminating labor because the patient does not conform to the usual lengths of latent, active, or second stages of labor. Falling outside of a numerical range does not document brain injury nor warrant an automatic clinical activity.

OBJECTIVES

At the conclusion of this chapter, the clinician should understand and be able to describe the following:

1. Labor terminology and the graphing of labor progress
2. General conduct of personnel in the labor and delivery room
    a. Obligations of the physician
    b. Use of monitoring
    c. Charting and documenting clinical events

CHART NOTES

Labor takes place over many hours during which the clinician is responsible for the patient's care. Complete chart notes in the course of labor enables the physician to review his or her earlier thoughts intelligently. It helps the clinician plan for and anticipate the progress of labor and recall what took place earlier. Memory of events considered important earlier in labor may not be as clear in the middle of the night. Years later when the record may be reviewed, a logical process for patient care may be more easily validated. Complete chart notes both facilitate and document the process of decision making. Chart notes, with date and time of day, document your attendance in the labor room.

LABOR GRAPHS

The labor graph should be constructed while labor is in progress (Figure 3.1). The graph presents a visual picture of labor, which helps the clinician understand patient progress and quickly determine the stage of labor. The labor graph allows obstetrical personnel to intervene promptly, if necessary. It replaces terms such as "good labor" or "poor progress" with a slope of cervical dilatation. A "good labor" in active phase should have an almost vertical slope of dilatation. The labor graph also allows the viewer to conceptualize the relationship between cervical dilatation and vertex descent. Descent and vertex engagement often occur late in labor. Many

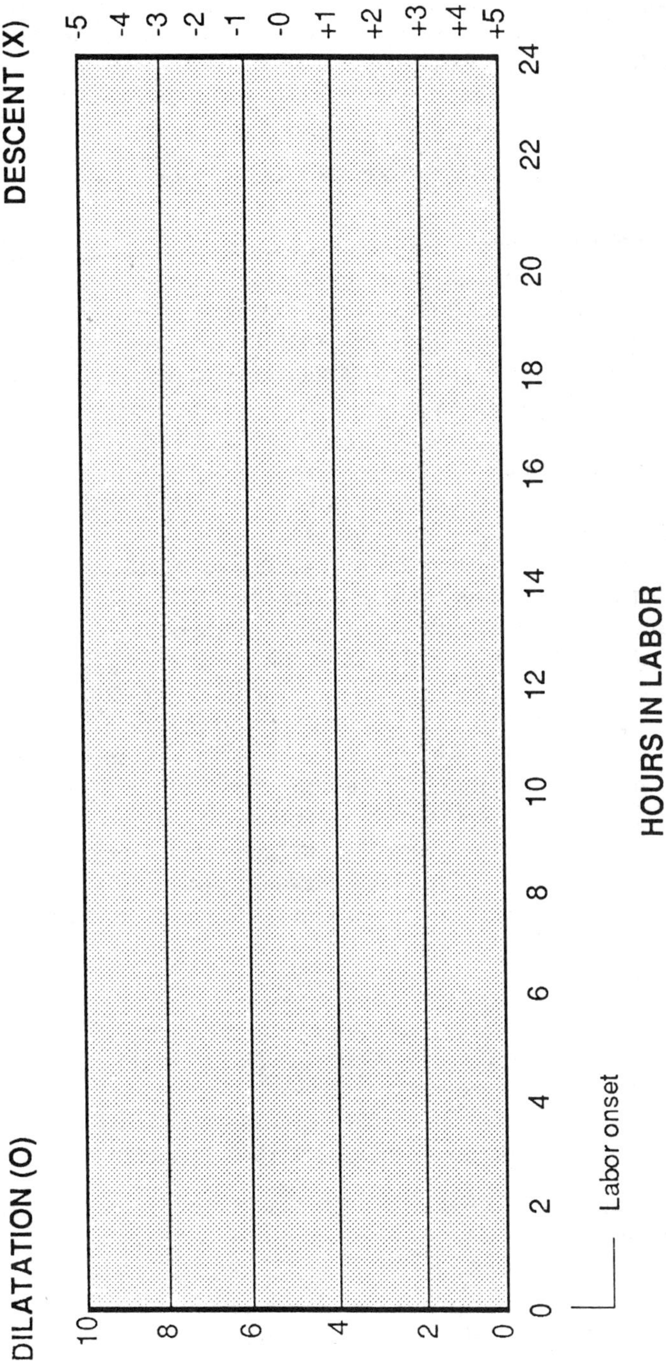
DILATATION (O)
DESCENT (X)
10
8
6
4
2
0
-5
-4
-3
-2
-1
-0
+1
+2
+3
+4
+5
0
2
4
6
8
10
12
14
16
18
20
22
24
Labor onset
HOURS IN LABOR

FIGURE 3–1

clinicians assume that active phase labor without vertex engagement is unusual, but in fact the converse is more correct and easily documented when graphing becomes ritual.

MEANING OF LABOR PROGRESS NUMBERS

The numbers defining progress in labor are guidelines and should be used with caution. By themselves, the standard deviations, means, and medians of large population studies do not indicate clinical or neurologic morbidity. For example, a person may be short and differ from the mean height of all people, or be two standard deviations shorter than the average person. Yet, although short, that individual is still a normal and healthy person. One may not infer that because of height the very short person is sick. A labor graph that documents a labor which "falls off" the Friedman curve and does not conform to the usual labor progress expected, does not mean that fetal damage has occurred or will occur.

Abnormal numbers in the latent or active phase of labor, such as prolongations, protractions, or arrests, are signals to assess *whether* interventions are needed. Alerted by the numbers and visual graph, the obstetrician understands that the patient's labor is not proceeding in the usual way and the labor warrants attention. Clinical care is improved by intervention at the correct time. When used appropriately, the labor numbers alert the physician of slow progress and he or she can then decipher the cause and intervene in a timely fashion. Deviations from standard graphical labor patterns have been used by some clinicians as a reason to terminate labor abruptly. When protractions or arrests are identified, the judgment of the physician should involve a choice of treatments that effect normal vaginal delivery. It is only after treatment choices have been considered that ending labor is acceptable.

GENERAL CONDUCT IN THE LABOR AND DELIVERY ROOM

Education for Childbirth and Support During Labor

Perhaps unnecessary to dwell upon, it has been established that a prepared mother manages the birthing experience more easily than an unprepared mother. Support personnel have historically been husbands. Today there is no reason why an alternative support person (friend, family member, or professional assistant) cannot assist the laboring mother. There is adequate information suggesting that labors are more easily managed, patients enjoy the experience more, and perhaps even the incidence of dystocia may be lowered in a more friendly birthing environment.[5]

Childbirth education is almost universally available. It is helpful if the materials being taught are similar to the procedures to which the patient will be exposed. There are times when physicians' procedures are not the same as those being taught in prenatal courses. It is the obligation of the medical staff (nurses, midwives, and physicians) to attempt to present a nonconfusing and consistent educational program. Ingrained in this is physician flexibility and patient choice.

It cannot be overemphasized that the full spectrum of labor information should be taught. An idealized version of the best of all outcomes may hinder a patient's adaptation if idealized labor does not take place. Some women may tolerate labor with little medication or anesthesia; some will not. The patient, suddenly confused by what, to her, is unexpected pain, may adapt to the labor poorly. Patient breakdown may influence early termination of labor. The prepared mother, educated to the full spectrum of potential labor events, including the pain of the contraction, is more easily supported during labor. It is the physician's obligation to understand what is being taught in the childbirth education courses.

EXAMPLE OF A POTENTIAL FOR CONFUSION IN TYPE OF LABOR ROOM SUPPORT

Two patients were overheard in the same physician's waiting room discussing their breathing exercises for labor. One patient described a series of five patterns she was being taught. The second was being taught a single breathing exercise for all of labor.

Comment

In the labor room, support for the patient after such varied educational programs will be most difficult if the information being taught is unknown to the support personnel.

PATIENT TREATMENT ROUTINES

Flexibility in treatment implies that no single pattern of care will apply to all patients.

EXAMPLE OF PATTERNED MEDICATION USE

Some physicians medicate all mothers using a fixed routine beginning at entry into the labor room, and supplemented every several hours thereafter.

Comment

This is a clinical care pattern best relegated to history. Judgment suggests that for different mothers in different labors, different patient medication programs may be needed. Normal patient care should be individualized.

EXAMPLE OF INDIVIDUALIZED CARE

At 4 cm of cervical dilation, a mother may request medication. In the low-risk healthy patient, this allows the clinician wide variability of choice. Patient choice should predominate.

Comment

The kind of pain relief used will be dictated by the labor progress the clinician perceives is taking place and by the patient's needs. The mother with the high vertex may be given 50 mg of meperidine intravenously to assist in relaxation between contractions. The mother with the well-engaged vertex may be offered an epidural block to remove all discomfort of contractions. The third mother may be tolerating the latent phase well and need no medication.

The average cervical dilatation for a patient to be ready to enter the labor and delivery room is near 4 cm.[2] Too early patient admissions should be avoided. Early labor may be better tolerated at home and require less medication.

PHYSICIAN PRESENCE DURING LABOR AND DELIVERY

Each physician will have different patterns for patient attention and for being present during the stages of labor. This will depend on the hospital environment, the support staff, and the patient. Whether the physician is present or not, responsibility for the patient remains with the patient's physician. That contract was established with the first antepartum visit and that responsibility cannot be transferred.

If Risk Is Present During Labor

In the presence of any risk to mother or fetus, the clinician should be present in order to make a personal evaluation. The clinician should continue to be easily available for consultation if an unexpected risk develops. If the physician cannot or chooses not to be present, a comparable alternate care provider must be chosen.

EXAMPLE OF ACUTE FETAL RISK AND PHYSICIAN PRESENCE

Telephone notification is received from the labor admitting nurse that there is a fetal heart pattern indicative of repetitive variable decelerations in a patient who is in early labor.

Comment

The obstetrician's attendance is required to review the materials until the situation is stabilized. If the physician chooses to have the situation evaluated by another responsible person while he/she is not physically present, that is a decision that should be most carefully made. As a responsible clinician, it is understood that while patient evaluation may be transferred, the responsibility for patient care (the results of the decision) is not transferable. If something goes wrong the responsibility remains with the patient's obstetrician.*

EXAMPLE OF CHRONIC FETAL RISK AND PHYSICIAN PRESENCE

The patient arrived in the labor screening area with ruptured membranes. Pea soup meconium stained amniotic fluid was described to the obstetrician by the examining nurse.

Comment

While the actual fetal risk for the release of that meconium may have taken place hours or days earlier, the condition should be evaluated at the bedside until a decision as to the severity of the problem is reached and a judgment concerning patient care is effected.

---

*While the care is described as being given by the individual physician, it is understood that in group practices the responsibility remains in the group, although at any one time assumed by an individual physician.

Can the obstetrician stay in an office in a building nearby, or an office connected to the hospital, or on the floor below the labor unit as the labor continues? That is a clinical judgment only the obstetrician can answer after seeing the patient. If the clinician has doubts, obviously the answer is to stay with the patient. Always write a timed and dated chart note describing your findings and impressions at the time of seeing the patient.

If Labor Is Normal

The clinician will rarely stay at the bedside continuously through labor. Some people may argue that the physician should always be present but the facts speak for themselves. The physician cannot always be there. The labor room environment and support system for patient care must be factors in the physician's decision to be present or not.

In the presence of a normal labor, "physician presence" has more latitude. Early in the latent phase of the labor of a vertex fetal presentation, greater choice exists. In contrast, with a breech presentation the situation should be managed differently.

Although stated facetiously, perhaps one of the major improvements in obstetrical patient care was the idea that adequate lounge and sleeping facilities should be available so that the obstetrician could be comfortable in the labor room environment.

Today, group practice appears to be replacing the solo practitioner. In these groups physicians are often assigned to labor rooms on a full-time basis. This constant attention is more "time" expensive, but good quality care is maintained. It is also often unavailable except in groups with large obstetrical services.

Because the physician has so frequently chosen not to stay at the bedside, nurses, midwives, and other labor partners have filled this void. There is little doubt that this personalized support relieves anxiety, makes the labor more tolerable, and may shorten the labor.[5] Sharing bedside support improves patient care.

Responsibility for Patient Care

It may be thought by some that the bedside care for the patient can be transferred to other persons such as nurses or resident physicians. In the event of a problem, it is the obstetrician's responsibility whether in the labor room, in the building next door, or at home. Responsibility is not transferrable.

CHART DOCUMENTATION: RECORD KEEPING

When charts are reviewed for hospital quality assurance programs, educational case discussions, research purposes, or courtroom appearances, all too often they show less than adequate physician's notes. In fact, far more care usually is given by physicians than is recorded in the medical chart. Nurses are trained to "chart" more frequently and completely than physicians. The physician must learn to chart appropriately. Notes, findings, and thoughts are needed and must be expressed in writing. It is embarrassing to have to write this in an educational format, but hospital chart review makes this deficiency clear. As mentioned earlier, the notes should be complete—dated and timed—and written soon after the evaluation.

Admission to Labor and Delivery: A First Evaluation

On admission to the labor room, a full evaluation is performed. This assessment should include a general history and physical evaluation written in the hospital chart. Statements should be made about the estimated size of the fetus, its pelvic position, the maternal phase of labor, and its quality. If there is deviation from the normal and expected findings, this should be noted.

Patient Plan Following the Admission Note (Table 3.1)

It is helpful to estimate what you anticipate in the course of the labor. Is a normal course of labor expected? By stating expectations, not only will this predictive process improve with experience, but the written record is established as a base for later patient care.

TABLE 3.1 Notes for Admission[a]

1. Date and time of writing note
2. Patient description of labor history
3. Significant historical data
4. General physical examination
5. Obstetrical examination
6. Evaluation of labor and prognosis

[a]Complete this note shortly after the examination.

EXAMPLE OF COMPLETION OF ADMISSION NOTE BY THE RESPONSIBLE PHYSICIAN

Someone else has already examined the patient and an admission note has been written for you by a resident or nurse. This note may be your first chart entry.

> 4/20/88, 1AM: The patient states her contractions began 7PM on 4/19. The abdominal examination confirms a vertex presentation with the back in the left side and vertex dipping into the pelvis. The estimated fetal weight is 7 lb. On vaginal examination the vertex is at station 3. The membranes are intact; the cervix is 3 cm dilated and 90% effaced. The patient is probably in the latent phase of labor. (Note: You must observe cervical dilatation to confirm labor.) I anticipate no problems. The patient has requested that no monitoring be performed unless necessary. The use of monitoring has been discussed during office visits, and the patient's request is accepted.

Comment

In the above example, the clinician's note did not include the patient's past history or physical examination. In this case, it was inferred that the information had already been obtained by others and read by the patient's responsible physician. It would be appropriate to state, "Admitting information reviewed and agreed with."

If no examination has taken place, the data should be obtained; a short note would include relevant historical information, vital signs, and pertinent physical findings. Most accreditation agencies request a complete history, including a social history and a physical examination.

The decision against electronic monitoring infers an adequate auscultation support system. In the normal patient, the use of electronic monitoring is a clinical judgment and need not be arbitrarily performed. There must, as noted, be adequate support to provide auscultation approximately every 30 minutes during latent phase labor, and each 15 minutes during active phase. The auscultated information should be charted.

Progress Notes

Later in labor additional written observations are helpful. Should these notes be written hourly? Probably not. Frequency of notation is determined by patient progress and the presence of normal or problem situations. Review the earlier notes. It is always helpful to read earlier thoughts.

Some clinician's have suggested that hourly vaginal examinations should be the rule. In latent labor this is not necessary. In active labor an hourly examination is more appropriate.

EXAMPLE OF A PROGRESS NOTE

> 4/20/88, 1PM: At 9AM the patient was 8 cm dilated with vertex at −3 station. Since that time this patient has made no progress. An arrest of

> cervical dilation and descent of the vertex in the active phase is present. On clinical examination, the patient's pelvis appears adequate for this fetus. Contractions are occurring each 4 minutes and are of poor quality. Oxytocin will be used to overcome this arrest of labor. Fetal monitoring has been without decelerations and with normal beat-to-beat variability.

Comment

Intervention could have occurred even earlier, often within 2 hours in a no-progress situation. However, differences in judgment allow for this flexibility in patient care. In other treatment choices, the patient could have been rested, medicated, or allowed to ambulate—choices dependent on patient needs. If in 1 to 2 hours no progress had occurred despite the use of oxytocin, your next note should complete the record, describing your thoughts and the reasons for your next decision. Note that the number of hours an arrest should be allowed to persist is not yet specified. Also note that the electronic fetal heart rate information was described as being without decelerations and with good beat-to-beat variability. This is a far more appropriate description than terms such as normal or abnormal which, to some clinicians, infer pathology. The heart rate tracing does not mean that there is brain abnormality. Its association with brain abnormality is extremely limited.

EXAMPLE OF CONTINUING PROGRESS NOTES

> 4/20, 3PM: No progress has been made for the past 3 hours despite adequate contractions stimulated with oxytocin. The fetal monitoring record remains normal. The cervix remains 8 to 9 cm. Moderate caput is present. The now molded vertex with caput is at S-2 (five station pelvis). A cesarean is to be performed for arrest in the active phase of labor.

Comment

Some practitioners might not have allowed the arrest to continue beyond 2 hours before the original intervention (oxytocin). Some might have medicated the patient. Others would have ended the oxytocin augmentation after 1 hour if progress did not take place. The final decision in this case was to perform a cesarean. Later in time, by reading the clinical notes, a quality assurance committee or an attorney would know the condition of the fetus during the arrest and why the decision was made. During the hours of patient care, the presence of the physician's notes enables the clinician to review the reasoning process. Two or 3 years after the birth, in the absence of complete notes, it will not be possible to reconstruct the process, and, if attempted, it may not be believed without a written record.

There is no specific time to end a trial of labor. In the presence of a normal pregnancy, normal monitoring, and absent meconium during labor would not cause criticism of this patient's care. In the presence of other risks, the clinician may have ended labor earlier. Electronic monitoring was needed as there was an other than usual labor pattern (an indication for monitoring), and because oxytocin was used (an indication for monitoring).

ELECTRONIC FETAL MONITORING

The availability of monitoring at the hospital where labor is planned, and the discussion of its use, should have taken place during the antenatal period. Although rarely recorded in charts, it is helpful to have *antenatal* and *intrapartal* notes documenting a discussion as to whether monitoring should be used.

The benefits of electronic fetal monitoring continues to be controversial in our medical society. In the low-risk patient, in the absence of intrapartal problems and the presence of adequate support persons for auscultation (listening each 30 minutes during latent phase, each 15 minutes during active phase), choice is available.

EXAMPLE OF DOCUMENTATION OF FETAL MONITORING REQUEST

Earlier during pregnancy, Mrs. Smith and I discussed the use of fetal monitoring. We discussed this again this evening in her labor room with her husband. They understand the reasons for monitoring use, including its value in some unpredictable labor problems such as occlusion of the umbilical cord. They prefer no use of electronic monitoring.

Comment

The antenatal record should document the discussions. Later, recall by the patient of monitoring discussions occurring only during a tension period in the labor room may be quite different.

Many hospitals have rules requiring electronic monitoring of all patients. Other hospitals allow flexibility in the absence of fetal risk. There are arguments to support each philosophy. There has been little change in knowledge about monitoring since the publication entitled *Antenatal Diagnosis: Intrapartum Fetal Distress* by the National Institutes of Health in 1979.[6] Therefore, choice for monitoring use is still available. Until the time comes when monitoring may take place so easily that it is neither cumbersome nor burdensome to patient and staff, and the use of the information is so clear that error in use of monitoring is lessened, it is preferable to offer a choice to the normal patient in labor.

THE HOSPITAL

Early in pregnancy the patient should be made aware of all of the hospital's capabilities for support. If a hospital exists in an environment where other hospitals are not accessible, patient choice of a hospital to labor in is obviously limited. In contrast, if several hospitals exist near enough to permit patient choice, and different levels of medical support are present at the adjacent hospitals, information should be given to the patient in order to assist her in making an informed choice.

Patient concerns may include the availability of scalp blood examinations, in-hospital presence of anesthesiologists, availability of emergency operating room facilities, and neonatal support systems. This information should be part of the childbirth educational program. An opportunity to visit the labor and delivery room environment and meet the nursing staff should be part of this educational experience.

PATIENT SENSITIVITY AND PATIENT INFORMATION

Although awareness of patient sensitivity is basic to clinical care, it cannot be overemphasized that respect for privacy, personal rights, and free exchange of information is expected. No longer is the physician allowed to introduce clinical care and expect treatment to be accepted without explanation. It is easier to exchange information before carrying out intervention rather than afterwards, especially if a complication may have occurred.

It is rare for a patient to demand an alternate medical care decision. As the physician, you are not giving up your right to give medical care by reviewing the problem. Rather, good judgment and sharing information is part of the process. However, no matter how the treatment is explained, the responsibility for the outcome will be the physician's.

Privacy and personal feelings in the labor room environment must be protected. Statements such as "Please," "Thank you," "May I come in," "May I examine you" (closing the door when you do), may be lost in a busy labor and delivery suite. Yet, long after the birth has occurred, many patients raise questions totally unexpected by the physician, but extremely important to the mother.

EXAMPLE OF PATIENT CHOICE IN A BREECH PRESENTATION

At term, a P3 G2 mother in latent labor with the cervix 4 cm dilated and at -2 station is informed that the fetus is in a frank breech presentation. A vertex presentation had been presumed during the antepartum period.

Comment

A discussion of choice for vaginal or cesarean birth should be initiated. In the situation where there is disagreement among physicians as to how the breech should be delivered, the patient should be informed of the variations in treatment philosophies. This is a classic situation where patient choice often resolves the question, and the physician often influences the outcome by the manner in which the information is presented.

Because of their concern about high cesarean birthrates, some physicians discuss potential problem situations at the onset of patient care. At the patient's request, dystocia, fetal distress, and previous cesareans are often reviewed prior to labor. Patient understanding of information presented in a non-tension-filled environment (antepartum) makes decisions regarding patient care during labor much easier.

EXAMPLE OF BIASING A PATIENT'S CHOICE

Mrs. Kelly is given all the information about the baby's breech position and patient choice, but when complications are discussed, Mrs. Kelly is told the baby's head may get trapped, and if that occurs, cerebral palsy and brain damage is a possibility.

Comment

That is no choice. Mrs. Kelly will respond, "I want a cesarean to protect my child." The patient decision, biased by the manner in which the physician introduced the information, will be for performing the cesarean. Yet, the patient must know the potential risks involved in each choice. It is not simple to discuss risk, which is possible but not common, and this is well understood by all clinicians.

EXAMPLE OF BIASING A PATIENT'S CHOICE

Mrs. Kelly is given all the information about the baby's breech position and the risks. In addition, she is also told that it is believed this baby will do as well when born by the vaginal birth route as by any alternative intervention.

Comment

This presents a different choice, but this, too, is not yet free from physician bias. This example more often will result in a vaginal delivery. The first example, with the inclusion of all potential specific fetal risks and little alternative to the cesarean, is perhaps why so many breech presentations are delivered by surgery.

Between these two examples, there must be a middle route of presenting the risks without exaggeration. When there is no absolute answer, it is a patient choice situation. The breech presentation is such an example.

EXAMPLE OF A SITUATION WHERE THERE SHOULD BE NO PATIENT CHOICE

A P1 G2 mother, at term, presents in labor actively bleeding bright red blood. About 600 cc of blood has been estimated to have been lost since the onset of contractions. Electronic fetal monitoring reveals repeated late decelerations following each contraction.

Comment

The patient is quickly informed of the need for a rapid evaluation to find the etiology of the hemorrhage. This situation still requires an information exchange, but, in contrast with the breech presentation, patient choice is not available. All necessary steps should be instituted to provide rapid resolution of the problem. The patient should not debate the issue, nor should she take away the physician's rights in emergency decisions. Exchange of the information in this case, takes place in a different manner.

Following situations such as this example, when decisions have been made rapidly, often in the midst of a medical crisis, it can induce patient emotional turmoil. Follow-up discussions during the postpartum period should take place. Lack of post-cesarean-delivery discussion frequently results in the patient requesting a repeat cesarean when given choice for a second trial of labor. The fear engendered by the first labor and surgery, and fetal concerns not understood or resolved, may lead to fear for recurrence. Why choose labor with this worry when the elective cesarean seems so simple?

LABOR AND DELIVERY ROOM ENVIRONMENT

The labor room environment can be emotionally supportive or disturbing. The sounds from adjacent laboring patients may be frightening. Physicians' conversations about labor-related issues (when not explained), or casual discussions about other patients or non-labor events may be perceived by the laboring mother in a very different frame of reference than by the speakers. Laughing over jokes, or even odors from foods cooked in a nearby microwave oven can be upsetting to the individual patient or her family.

EXAMPLE OF INFORMATION REQUESTED LONG AFTER LABOR

One year following a cesarean delivery because of hypertensive encephalopathy, a mother requested an opportunity to return to the labor and recovery rooms. This came as a surprise to the physician who began to elucidate more information relating to this request.

Comment

On further questioning, the physician learned that the patient had no recollection of the 48-hour period during which she had been critically ill. One year later she still had recurring nightmares about what might have taken place during the time she was mentally obtunded. She wished to see the rooms and people she could not remember.

EXAMPLE OF MISUNDERSTANDING A HALLWAY DISCUSSION

A discussion of the fetal distress which was occurring in patient A's labor took place outside the doorway of patient B's room. Patient B heard the conversation and concluded that this "fetal distress" referred to her son.

Comment

Despite a normal labor and delivery, the mother raised her child with the internalized fears that he was different and needed more help and understanding because he had incurred fetal distress. Her son was always referred to as her "sick child." No one realized that she had heard the adjacent patient's problems being discussed by the staff. The obstetrician learned of her fears years later during a casual conversation taking place at an annual check-up. Review of her labor records confirmed that there had been no fetal distress.

FETAL DISTRESS AND EMERGENCY CESAREAN

In contrast to an imagined problem, if a problem such as fetal distress should occur, the meaning of fetal distress should be discussed with the patient again after the completion of labor.

In the postoperative period, to the patient, the term fetal distress implies risk and trauma. The actions taken during labor to evaluate and avoid a problem often remove control of labor from the patient to the medical personnel. The patient is told to turn from one side to the other. Suddenly, an oxygen mask is placed over her nose and mouth. In the extreme case, the abdomen is rapidly shaved, a Foley catheter inserted, and she is rolled into a new room—the operating room. Among new persons, often without her husband, the patient is rapidly placed under anesthesia. It is little wonder that many patients are physically and psychologically traumatized by labor events and are determined not to undergo labor again.

It should be pointed out that a fetal heart rate recording described as fetal distress does not necessarily result in later developmental abnormality. It is an indication that a period of increased observation is needed to avoid increasing fetal risk. Fetal distress may mean fetal risk; it infrequently means fetal damage. Fetal distress concerning a patient should not be discussed where a second patient may listen. In labors when the diagnosis of fetal distress leads to surgery, the parents need a complete discussion of the events that took place, and when possible, reassured that the infant's future is optimistic. In addition, an explanation of the events that took place prior to the cesarean is of value. This should take place on several occasions during the postpartum period and repeated at the 6-week visit. Lack of information creates more fear than explained problems.

SUMMARY

1. The Friedman labor definitions will be used throughout this text.
2. Definitions are guides to interventions and not rules which must be adhered to.
3. Active plotting of labor graphs will allow for improved clinical evaluation and education of all personnel.
4. The conduct of all labor room personnel and the physical and emotional support systems for patients during labor are integral parts of patient care.
5. In the presence of fetal risk, or until the fetal risk is evaluated, the obstetrician should be with the patient.
6. Electronic fetal monitoring should be used with the risk patient and offered to the normal patient.
7. Admission and progress notes should be written by the clinician as they are helpful during patient care and invaluable for later review.
8. Sensitivity to patient needs and a supportive labor room environment are also a physician's responsibility.

REFERENCES

1. Friedman EA: Labor: Clinical Evaluation and Management, ed 2. New York, Appleton-Century-Crofts, 1978.
2. Peisner DB, Rosen MG: The latent phase of labor in normal patients: a reassessment. Obstet Gynecol 1985; 66:644–648.
3. Peisner DB, Rosen MG: Transition from latent to active labor. Obstet Gynecol 1986; 68:448–500.
4. Rosen MG, Peisner DB: Effect of amniotic membrane rupture on length of labor. Obstet Gynecol 1987; 70:604–607.
5. Sosa R, Kennell J, Klaus M, Robertson S, Urrutia J: The effect of a supportive companion on perinatal problems, length of labor, and mother–infant interaction. N Engl J Med 1980; 303:597–600.
6. Antenatal Diagnosis: Intrapartum Fetal Distress, publication 79–1973. Bethesda, MD, National Institutes of Health, 1979.

Chapter 4

The Clinical Examination

OVERVIEW

The clinical examination includes the patient's general history and a physical examination, performed for all patients upon admission to the hospital, as well as the obstetrical examination. Because the laboring patient has usually been seen and examined completely during the previous year, the contents of the general history and physical examination may be condensed, introducing only pertinent or new information. In contrast, the obstetrical examination is too often neglected or simplified. A complete obstetrical examination, including an abdominal examination and clinical pelvimetry, should be performed.

OBJECTIVES

At this conclusion of this chapter, the clinician should recognize the need for the following:

1. Documentation of important historical information and general physical findings of patients in labor
2. A complete obstetrical examination to evaluate the patient and plan for the completion of labor
   a. Abdominal examination
   b. Vaginal examination
   c. Clinical pelvimetry

3. Ultrasonography as a supportive laboratory test for the clinical examination
4. The limitations of x-ray and clinical pelvimetry

GENERAL HISTORY AND PHYSICAL EXAMINATION

Overemphasis on technology often results in destruction of the sensitive relationship between the clinician and patient early in labor. Today it is a unique situation to be able to examine a patient in early labor without the presence of an already in-place monitoring system covering her abdomen. It is not unusual to have the pelvic examination followed by abdominal ultrasonography without complete patient evaluation ever taking place.

Although the patient in labor has already undergone a thorough history and physical examination, the process must be respected. A review of the patient's interval history should take place; i.e., recent illness, medications, and diet. Unusual allergies or illness should then be reconfirmed and drug use recorded in the chart note. A general physical examination including vital signs, heart and lung evaluations, mental acuity, presence of drugs, and neurologic reflexes should take place. If the physical examination is normal, this should be noted, as well as all positive findings.

OBSTETRICAL EVALUATION

Observation

Observe the patient and look at her abdomen. By the time many clinicians see their patients in labor, the patients' abdomens are covered with various external belts. It is quite helpful to look at the maternal abdomen and begin to determine the following:

1. Fetal size: A speculation, but it can be an early warning of a large or small fetus.
2. Fetal lie: Long before ultrasonography is used, an oblique or transverse lie can be suspected by looking at the abdomen. An unusual presentation can be confirmed with ultrasonography after the physical examination is completed.
3. Fetal position: Before the manual abdominal examination is performed, there should be an attempt to visualize on which side the fetal back lies. When medical students or residents are asked to look at the maternal abdomen of a seventh or eighth month patient and point to the side the fetal back is on, they inevitably choose the round side rather

than the straight side. The back, when it can be seen in late pregnancy, is the straight side of the maternal abdomen; the arms and legs produce the round convexity.

EXAMPLE OF AN ABDOMINAL EXAMINATION COMPLIMENTING THE VAGINAL EXAMINATION

A primigravid woman at 38 weeks of gestation was in the active phase of labor, 6 cm dilated with vertex S-3. Abdominal observation noted the straight side was on the left and the round side on the right (therefore, the back was on the left side). Following vaginal examination, the examiner was uncertain if the vertex was right occiput anterior (ROA) or left occiput posterior (LOP) as the head was not well flexed and the fontanels could not be easily felt.

Comment

The answer was straightforward. Knowing that the fetal back was on the left side following the clinical examination would have eliminated the confusion. In a vertex presentation, the back and the occiput are on the same side. This finding would also allow the clinician to anticipate a longer time to delivery as it usually takes more time for the occiput posterior fetus to rotate and descend.

Similarly, "looking" while a patient is bearing down during the second stage of labor is also helpful.

EXAMPLE OF VISUALIZING VAGINAL DILATION DURING STAGE OF LABOR

A G3 P2 mother with a fully dilated cervix and vertex at S+2 (five stations to the pelvis) was voluntarily pushing with each contraction. At the height of each pushing effort, everyone was anticipating caput. It was obvious that the labia were separating during her expulsive efforts. However, there was no caput visible. In this circumstance even without a vaginal digital examination, using your "observation," you would know a wider diameter of the fetal vertex is presenting. Thus, either a larger vertex or an occiput transverse or posterior is on its way. The larger diameters of the presenting vertex in these situations distend the labia earlier, before caput is visible. The birth will take longer until descent, either with or without rotation, takes place, and then crowning will be seen.

Palpate the Abdomen: The Four Maneuvers of Leopold

1. Palpate the fundus and estimate its height. The height of the fundus as "weighed" by the examiner's hands is still a good estimator of fetal size. This is always modified by whether or not membranes are ruptured, by

the patient's size, or the fetal lie. The examination is least accurate in the presence of unusual fetal positions, or at the extremes of fetal weight.

If there is uncertainty as to whether the fetal part in the fundus is the breech, continue gently holding the fundus with one or both hands for several moments. Holding on to the breech is often associated with kicking or palpable movements of the fetal extremities which are not felt with the vertex. Fetal heart deceleration associated with pressure or squeezing on the vertex has not been as helpful. In many labor rooms the ultrasound machine can and should be used as needed. However, the clinical examination still has its place.

2. The second movement of Leopold will be facilitated by the impression of fetal lie already in mind from earlier observations and palpations. While still facing the maternal head, run both hands along the sides of the uterus. Palpation of the back will be facilitated by earlier impressions of visualizing the straight side and the often moving extremities on the opposite side.
3. Still facing the patient's head, grasp the presenting part and attempt to move it. It may be immovable and well fixed in the pelvis (possibly engaged) or easily movable (probably not engaged). This is an uncomfortable procedure for the patient. Be gentle in trying to reach low enough behind the pubic symphysis to complete this maneuver.
4. Turn towards the patient's feet and with both hands moving along the sides of the vertex, note whether the examining hands begin to converge (unengaged as the top of the head is reached) or diverge (possibly engaged). In the uncommon face presentation, the hyperextended head may be palpated on the same side as the back. If the abdominal examination is not performed before the vaginal examination it is usually neglected. Many clinicians have incorrectly estimated vaginal position of the vertex because they did not pursue a complete clinical examination.

The above discussion may appear almost insignificant. However, there is no obstetrician who at times has not been uncertain as to fetal vertex position. Use everything that is available; that is the clinical art of obstetrics.

General Vaginal Examination

This examination is performed with sterile gloves and without additional washing or preparation of the perineum, which has never been documented as increasing sterility of the exam. The vaginal examination is the final step in documenting the fetal position and predicting the progress of the labor. It is for the prediction of the outcome of the labor that these examinations are performed.

Clinical pelvimetry, or clinical measurements of the pelvis, are not usually performed as routine labor examinations. Clinical pelvimetry is described as a potential need and is usually performed at the first antenatal visit. During labor the patient is uncomfortable, pelvic muscle relaxation is not attainable, and the vertex may be in the way of the clinician's attempts to measure the diagonal conjugate.

Fundal pressure may allow an estimate of how easily the vertex may descend into the pelvis later. If the vertex descends with fundal pressure, and perhaps reaches or exceeds the levels of the ischial spines, fetal and pelvic size should not be an anticipated problem. This maneuver is a guide though, not an absolute answer.

During the later vaginal examination, an estimate should be made of how much room there is in the pelvis by noting space around the vertex and in the hollow of the sacrum. The examination should be performed while thinking in terms of pelvic capacity. Is the pelvis large enough? Is there room around the head? Does the head descend? If the examination is performed only to measure cervical dilatation and assess vertex station, then the physician may believe—as others have suggested—that pelvic assessment is useless.

Vaginal Examination of the Cervix and Presenting Part

The vaginal examination during labor should also disclose cervical effacement, dilatation, the presenting part and its position, and the relationship of the presenting part to the ischial spines.

Cervical effacement is measured by percentages or gross estimates, and will give important information as to labor length. A 40% or 50% thick cervix foreshadows a longer labor. A cervix almost 100% effaced foreshadows much shorter labor.

Cervical dilatation is usually estimated and needs little comment. It is slow in rate of dilatation during latent phase, and more rapid in active phase. Is the cervix anterior or posterior? If the cervix is well behind or posterior, anticipate a longer time for dilatation.

Vertex position is next evaluated. Think of the position of the fontanels. Identifying their location allows estimates of flexion and asynclitism. Is the vertex well flexed (the posterior fontanel is the key), hyperextended (the anterior fontanel is palpated more easily), or in midposition (neither fontanel predominates; both must be reached for)? A poorly flexed vertex infers that larger diameters of the vertex are presenting. It will take more labor time and work to complete the process.

Sutures of the vertex, coordinated with the fontanels, supplement the estimate of flexion of the vertex and the identification of the fontanels. The sagittal suture also adds information as to lateral flexion or asynclitism. For example, in a vertex with occiput transverse, a posterior or "U" position of the sagittal suture will suggest to the examiner that the anterior parietal bone is presenting.

Molding and caput of the presenting part are also important clinical indicators of what is expected in the labor. At times caput may be present early in labor through a partially dilated cervix, particularly when membranes are ruptured. Molding connotes that the diameters of the vertex are changing in the fetal attempt to traverse the pelvis. Molding may take place above the ischial spines, at higher pelvic stations in longer labors, or below the ischial spines after engagement during vaginal dilatation, when descent of the vertex has been more rapid or has occurred earlier. In general, in long labors molding will take place at higher stations, and in short labors time may be needed for the vertex to mold in order to traverse the vagina. Molding and caput, when felt during a difficult, active, or second stage of labor, suggests that the vertex is higher in the pelvis than it feels by palpation. In a protracted active phase or a slow vertex descent during the second stage, the vertex feels lower than it actually is. Do not focus on the increasing caput and molding of the fetal vertex with progress in descent.

EXAMPLE OF CONFUSION IN ESTIMATING PELVIC STATION

A primigravid patient was experiencing a delay in descent during the second stage of labor. After 3 hours of full dilatation, the vertex, which had been at S+1 at 5 PM, was felt to be at S+2 (five positive stations to the pelvis) at 8 PM, with an OP presentation.

Comment

Despite the station change, progress may still be arrested. The palpated descent may be increased molding and caput. The vertex is longer but the widest diameters are not lower. In an emergency and the need to deliver this fetus rapidly, be concerned that this delivery may be more difficult than the position that the vertex suggests. The vertex may truly be comparable to a station 0 or even unengaged. Clinical events and judgment as to birth route dictate your next acts, but cesarean rather than midforceps or vacuum extraction should be carefully considered.

Stations of the Pelvis

Generally use five stations to define the depth of the pelvis. Estimate engagement at station 0 to +1 with crowning at station +5. Some clinicians use three stations instead of five. Use of the same descriptive language would be helpful. The five stations are estimated in centimeters. These estimates become important in considering the application of forceps and the later discussion of how difficult the forceps are.

As noted before, some clinicians use fundal pressure to determine whether the presenting part dips into the pelvis or between the ischial spines and to predict adequate pelvic capacity. Descent often takes place late in labor for the primipara, and even more commonly takes place late in active or second stage for the multipara.

High stations of the presenting part in early labor foreshadow longer labors, but do not usually predict pelvic capacity. In latent labor findings, a station of S-4 rarely foreshadows "dystocia." Cesareans performed in latent phase labor for dystocia result from inaccurate estimates of pelvic capacity by the physician. The cervix needs to dilate; then descent tests the pelvis. Because estimates of pelvic capacity are always speculative, and because labor is not harmful, time to observe dilation and descent should be used before the labor is ended. In most instances, cervical dilatation will proceed whether or not descent takes place.

Referring back to Chapter 3, the initial admission and progress notes should include an obstetrical examination. The obstetrical examination should include the description of cervix and evaluation of the presenting part within the pelvis, as noted in Table 4.1.

CLINICAL PELVIMETRY

Today few clinicians can describe the anatomy of the pelvis with its four bones, including the sacrum, the coccyx, and the two innominate bones (also known as the ilium, the ischium, and the pubis) and the pelvis lying above the iliopectineal line, with its muscular insertions (iliac muscles) running into the bony pelvis below it. For a more complete review of

TABLE 4.1 Obstetrical Examination

1. Dilatation of cervix (also its *position*: anterior, posterior, etc)
2. Effacement of cervix (stated in percentage)
3. Presenting part (vertex, breech, other)
4. Position of fontanel (if both cannot be felt, think of the reason) When the head is not well flexed, a longer labor may be anticipated. Full flexion and extension must occur prior to most term births.
5. Station of presenting part in pelvis (if the spines are prominent, note this) Use five positive and five negative stations of antepartum care, and, when possible, during labor if progress is not satisfactory.

anatomy of the pelvis one may refer to the older anatomy texts by Ullery and Castalleo[1] or a more current volume of *Williams Obstetrics.*[2]

Measuring Pelvic Capacity

In contrast to defining bones and muscle insertions, which are of interest but have little practical application, the length of the diagonal conjugate, the size of the sacrosciatic notch, the shape of the sacrum, the prominence of the ischial spines, and the splay of the pelvic side walls convey useful information and should be measured at the onset of labor.

Estimating the diagonal conjugate is still a useful measurement. The term "estimate" is used with the understanding that the distance from sacral promontory to the underside of the symphysis pubis, as defined by the distance from your examining fingertip at the promontory, is stated to be about or greater than 11.5 cm. Usually, this measurement is adequate or longer than the examiner's finger may reach. If frequently performed on all patients, the repeated estimation of the diagonal conjugate allows the clinician to gain an experience estimating, not only possible inlet capacity, but also, as the finger traverses the hollow of the sacrum, the shape of the sacrum.

Can the head fit into the curve of the sacrum? This may be inferred if the sacrum is flat or knobby, thereby partially occluding the midplane and keeping the vertex high.

Are the spines so prominent that the vertex must rotate to an AP or oblique diameter before engagement can take place? Prominent spines suggest that a diameter other than the transverse diameter is necessary for engagement to take place.

Is the sacrosciatic notch wide? If so, expect more room in the posterior sagittal plane of the pelvis. The sacrosciatic notch is measured by moving the examining finger from the ischial spines, back along the sacrospinous ligament towards the sacrum. Once again, only after repeated attempts to make this estimate will the clinician gain sufficient experience to estimate size. In this case, the sacrosciatic notch is usually estimated to be between two- and three-finger-breadths (Fb) wide. A narrow ligament (<2Fb) suggests a high arch with little space in the posterior aspect of the pelvis. A wide arch (>3Fb) suggests a large posterior pelvis with more room for the vertex in this area of the pelvis.

It is difficult to estimate the pelvic sidewalls as the patient's muscle tensions often confuse the measurement. It is better measured during the patient's initial antepartum visit rather than during labor. In palpating the pelvic sidewalls, involuntary patient muscle contractions give the impression that the bony walls are convergent. In your mental picture of the pelvis, attempt to separate the muscle tension from the true convergent pelvis, which is quite uncommon.

A complete examination, including the above-mentioned measurements (diagonal conjugate, sacrosciatic notch, ischial spines, sacrum) along with the clinical estimate of what may be expected for the labor, allows the clinician to estimate labor length. While these estimates may be inaccurate or change as labor progresses, they act as signposts along the way and encourage reevaluation and earlier intervention.

In a pregnancy following a cesarean for dystocia, vaginally born siblings are often larger than their cesarean born predecessors. Therefore, it becomes apparent that despite the best clinical estimates, prediction for outcome will be only a first step towards a test of the pelvis with a trial of labor.

X-RAY PELVIMETRY

Whether or not to order x-ray pelvimetry always arouses debate. It would appear that the law courts have reintroduced the dilemma. The dilemma is that in the absence of absolute pelvic contracture the presenting part will flex, bend, mold, and work its way through this irregular passageway. Irrespective of clinical measurements, delivery will take place. X-ray pelvimetry is not needed. The x-ray measurements are only estimates, the numbers are far from exact. Because x-ray pelvimetry is infrequently used, both the persons taking the films and those reading the films confound the issues even further with their lack of knowledge. X-ray pelvimetry does not allow us to predict labor outcome. Obstetrical care has changed since the statement by Thoms[3] in the preface to his text on pelvimetry, that during the previous 25 years all patients in labor in the clinical service at the Yale–New Haven Hospital had undergone an x-ray exam on admission.

Rarely perform x-ray pelvimetry for the vertex presentation. This examination may be performed for the breech presentation for two reasons. The first reason is to confirm vertex flexion and absence of congenital anomalies, which can also be confirmed by ultrasonography or a flat x-ray film of the abdomen. The second reason is that after a difficult breech delivery, in the absence of an x-ray pelvimetry examination, the physician is always asked why x-ray pelvimetry was not obtained.

There is still not sufficient data on the use of computerized tomography, with or without ultrasonography of the vertex, to determine its usefulness. Until prospective controlled predictive studies are performed, the tests will lack validity. In the end it is the ability of the vertex to flex, mold, descend, and rotate through an irregular bone and muscle passageway which will determine whether the pelvis has adequate capacity.

SUMMARY

1. The general history and physical examination, although shortened because of previous examinations, should be reviewed at labor onset.
2. The obstetrical clinical evaluation consists of:

   a. Observing the abdomen
   b. Palpating the abdomen
   c. Estimating cervical dilatation and vertex position
   d. Clinical pelvimetry

3. Taken alone, each physical diagnostic task has limited value, but performed as a complete unit, adequate estimates of fetal size and pelvic capacity allow for more accurate predictions of labor length and labor outcome.
4. Clinical mensuration of the pelvis is best performed early in pregnancy, and cannot be used as an absolute predictor of successful or unsuccessful vaginal birth.
5. X-ray pelvimetry adds little to labor management or estimates of pelvic capacity.

REFERENCES

1. Ullery JC, Castalleo MA: Obstetrics Mechanisms and Their Management. Philadelphia, FA Davis, 1957.
2. Pritchard JA, MacDonald PC, Gant NF: Williams Obstetrics, ed 17. Norwalk, CT, Appleton-Century-Crofts, 1985, p 11.
3. Thoms H: Pelvimetry. New York, Hoeber-Harper, 1956, Preface p 9.

Chapter 5

The Latent Phase of Labor

OVERVIEW

In Chapters 5 through 9, the latent and active phases and the second stage of labor will be reviewed. Dystocia is presented separately in Chapter 10. In fact, there is overlap between phases and stages of labor and treatments of patients. Often, many of the same interventions are used in latent and active labor. There is additional overlap in discussing dystocia as a separate entity from labor patterns and their treatments. This reiterative process is used to present simple, repeated guidelines for clinical judgment in order to understand the reasons for clinical care.

In latent phase labor, indications for cesarean, such as poor progress, cephalopelvic disproportion, or dystocia are inaccurate. The data for making those decisions is not available. Later, in active phase or second stage of labor, when length of labor may be accurately predicted, length of time to delivery will modify this position.

During latent phase, labor decisions for terminating labor should, with rare exceptions, be based on urgent maternal or fetal indications. In the presence of fetal distress, the labor may be surgically terminated. Regardless of labor stage, in the presence of maternal hemorrhage, both maternal and fetal indications take precedence. Obviously, the degree of fetal or maternal distress will modify these clinical judgments.

OBJECTIVES

At the conclusion of this chapter, the clinician should be able to:

1. Define latent phase labor

2. Diagnose the many factors affecting latent phase labor
3. Describe management guidelines for latent phase labor
4. Lower the incidence of cesareans in latent phase labor

LATENT LABOR DEFINED

Contractions and Latent Phase Onset

Latent labor onset is defined as the point at which the mother perceives regular contractions. To be certain, latent phase labor onset must be followed by cervical dilatation as observed by the clinician.[1] Other clinicians suggest that labor onset would be more accurately defined by observed cervical dilatation after the patient arrives at the hospital.[2] Neither of these definitions defines physiology or pathology and are arguable. Either definition is acceptable as long as there is understanding among peers as to which system is used. In this text onset of labor is understood to begin with maternal perceptions of regular contractions.

The clinical problem is to determine whether (or not) the patient is in labor. That question can only be answered by observing cervical dilation which separates labor from false labor.

In earlier studies at Cleveland Metropolitan General Hospital[3,4] latent phase labor lengths (in hours) were derived from time of onset of contractions, as noted by the patient, and compared with the Friedman data which accepts a similar definition. The results were remarkably similar.

In addition to the time of contraction onset, latent labor must be characterized by observed cervical dilatation. No matter how long contractions have been occurring, how frequently they may be felt or palpated by staff, or visualized on a tocograph, labor cannot be characterized with certainty by uterine contractions alone. Dilatation must take place. An exception to that rule is extremely uncommon.

EXAMPLE OF DIFFICULTY IN DETERMINING LABOR ONSET

On arrival at the hospital, a PO G1 patient was experiencing extremely painful contractions every 2 minutes. As noted on the tocograph, the contractions were bell shaped with high peaks and poor return to the baseline. The vertex was floating; the cervix was 1 to 2 cm dilated in posterior position and 50% effaced. The fetal heart recording was normal. Diagnosis of possible placental abruption had been considered because of the severe maternal discomfort. Since there was no fetal distress, the patient was observed for the next 2 hours with the obstetrician sitting at the bedside.

Comment

The diagnosis of possible abruption was later replaced by the diagnosis of false labor after the obstetrician sat at the bedside of the patient. With reassurance and maternal support (which was badly needed by the tense patient), the contractions changed in frequency and became more widely spaced, finally occurring about one each 10 to 15 minutes. The patient soon fell asleep. Five hours later a decision was made to induce the patient who now had no contractions. In reviewing the previous events, it was felt that the patient was experiencing false labor.

No matter how well contractions may appear on the monitoring printout, contractions without dilatation cannot be equated with labor. In this unusual example the physician's presence at the bedside created a change in maternal anxiety and the disappearance of uterine contractions. At first, all would have agreed the patient was in labor and fetal risk from a possible abruption was present.

Onset of Dilatation

Although regular contractions may signal onset of the latent phase of labor, at the time contractions begin, neither patient nor physician can be certain that true labor is beginning. O'Driscoll and Meager[2] noted that in labor room evaluations of mothers with cervices dilated less than 4 cm, 10% of the patients were sent home because the diagnosis of active labor could not be confirmed.[4] One half of these patients soon returned in active labor, confirming that it is better for the patient to experience early labor at home. For the remainder, the diagnosis of false labor was correct. O'Driscoll and Meager did not feel that taking more time to estimate whether labor had begun prior to initiating active labor management was an important risk to mother or fetus. The study also demonstrates that even experienced clinicians have difficulty making the diagnosis of true or active labor.

EXAMPLE OF INDUCTION DURING POSSIBLE LATENT PHASE LABOR (FIGURE 5.1)

A primigravida at 38 weeks of gestation appeared in the screening area for the third successive night. Because of her emotional distress, an induction of labor with oxytocin was attempted. On admission, the cervix was 1 to 2 cm dilated, 50% effaced, in midposition, with vertex at S-3. The fetus appeared normal in size. Eighteen hours after the oxytocin infusion was begun, the cervix was 3 cm dilated. For the first time it was felt that the patient was in labor (latent phase).

Comment

In this patient it was necessary to induce labor in less than favorable circumstances. As was predictable by the only partially effaced cervix, a long latent phase should have been anticipated. It is this clinical situation which leads to patient and physician exhaustion and increased cesarean rates. Eventually, if allowed to progress, this exhausted patient will tolerate active and second stage labor even less well than the present situation. Once again, interventions such as cesareans and forcep use will occur more frequently. As seen in Figure 5.1, this looks like a problem labor, but it is only a long latent phase induction.

An alternate treatment could have been the use of adequate amounts of morphine subcutaneously, allowing the patient to sleep in the hospital overnight. Morphine or demerol rather than a barbiturate is suggested as pain was part of the clinical picture.

In general, the patient in early latent phase of labor belongs at home. In the Cleveland study less than 16.2% of normal laboring patients were admitted with admission exams of less than 3 cm cervical dilatation.[3] The key for diagnosis of latent phase labor is observed dilatation. As Hendricks et al[5] has stated, the cervix may dilate several weeks before labor begins. Thus, the antepartum nullipara or multipara with cervix dilated at 1 to 2 cm is not uncommon, and 3 to 4 cm is not rare. In Table 5.1, note that *at the time of admission for labor* the median dilation for nulliparous patients was 4 to 5 cm. If much of the latent phase of labor is spent at home, labor appears shorter to both mother and obstetrician.

TABLE 5.1 Dilatation of Patients on Admission[a]

Dilatation (cm)	% of patients
1	0
2	3.4
3	12.8
4	22.7
5	22.7
6	13.6
7	9.7
8	5.4
9	4.0
10	1.4
Complete	4.3
	100

[a]Normal patients with normal labors.
Modified from Ref. 3.

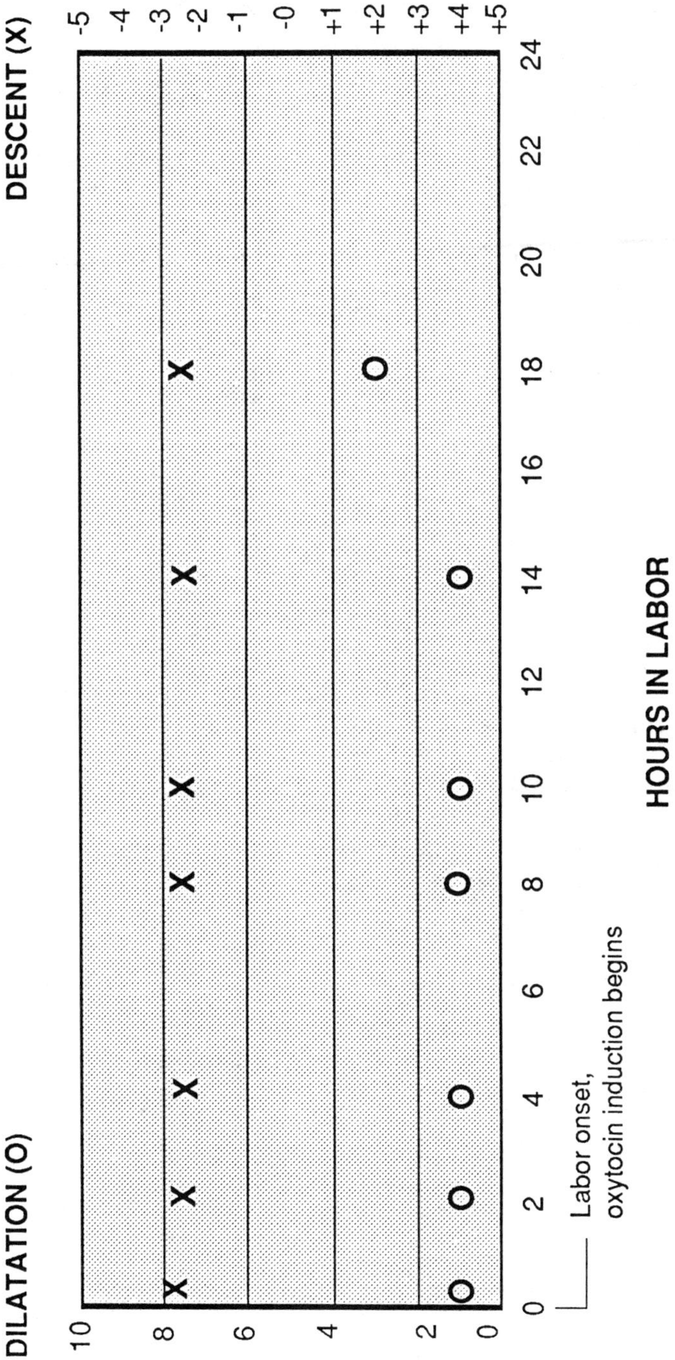
DILATATION (O)
DESCENT (X)
10
8
6
4
2
0
-5
-4
-3
-2
-1
-0
+1
+2
+3
+4
+5
0
2
4
6
8
10
12
14
16
18
20
22
24
Labor onset,
oxytocin induction begins
HOURS IN LABOR

FIGURE 5.1

End of Latent Phase—Onset of Active Phase

The Friedman criteria for entry into the active phase of labor are acceptable standards. The nullipara accelerates to or exceeds a cervical dilatation rate of 1.2 cm/h. The multipara progresses at 1.5 cm/h in active labor. Understand that this rate of cervical dilatation does not start at a specific dilatation. In the analysis of latent labor, 29% of patients reached 5 cm of dilatation before their dilatation rates conformed to the Friedman dilatation ratio.[4] Conversely, other patients dilated more rapidly and had active labor phase cervical dilation rates as early as 3 cm of cervical dilatation.

For simplicity, if at term, with uterine contractions appearing in a laborlike pattern with observed cervical dilatation, and when the active phase rate of cervical dilation is not already documented, all patients should be classified as "in active labor" when at 5 cm of dilatation. If progressive cervical dilatation is not present at 5 cm, the obstetrician must begin to think of treatment. Questions should be asked such as why orderly dilatation has not occurred and what obstetrical interventions should be used to improve progress in labor.

Rather than set an arbitrary length to latent phase of labor, Table 5.2 may be used to document mean latent labor duration percentage of patients at dilations varying from 0 to 5 cm.[3] These average lengths of latent phase may guide the clinician to intervene when these limits are passed. In Friedman's descriptions, a prolonged latent phase is greater than 20 hours for the nulligravida and greater than 14 hours for the primigravida.[6] Neither number predicts abnormality of the active phase nor increased fetal morbidity, they simply state that 90% of all women (nullipara or multipara) will have entered active labor by the end of the mean time period, according to dilatation at admission. From the Cleveland Metropolitan General Hospital data,[3] the mean length of latent labor for all patients was 6 hours and 49 minutes. However, this was a low-risk, normal population with amniotic membranes intact at labor onset.

In summary, the latent phase of labor ends at 5 cm dilatation or earlier

TABLE 5.2 Mean Latent Labor Duration[a]

Admission dilatation (cm)	Mean h: min
0–2	9 h 27 min
2–3	7 h 46 min
3–5	5 h 22 min

[a]From Ref. 3.

if the rate of dilatation equals or exceeds 1.2 cm/h for the nullipara, or at 1.5 cm/h for the multipara. Early latent phase is best treated at home. Patients and physicians appear to perform better if early latent phase of labor is not spent in a labor room. The onset of latent phase labor may only be judged in retrospect after cervical dilation has been observed.

Ruptured Membranes and Latent Phase Labor

In the presence of ruptured membranes, the patient is often admitted to the hospital. The question of prolapse of the umbilical cord and consequent fetal death is quite rare, and is about 1 per 2,000 live births in term infants during labor.[7] This figure was obtained prior to the era of monitoring and refers to *all* of labor, not only the situation of membrane rupture prior to labor.

Treatment following rupture of membranes without labor onset is not yet standardized. At term with an inducible cervix (or after the 34th week at the Sloane Hospital for Women of the Presbyterian Hospital in New York City) most clinicians would induce the labor. If the cervix is not easily inducible, almost any pattern of care has been recorded in the literature from no induction to induction at varying time intervals. Data proving efficacy for one consistent mode of treatment is not available. Cord prolapse and infections are the major concerns.

In the fetus prior to 35 weeks of gestation varied modes of treatment have been proposed with no single program being accepted. In the low-birth-weight fetus, more clinicians tend to await labor onset rather than induce with oxytocin. In this population infection is more morbid. All patients with ruptured membranes prior to labor onset should have cervical cultures to rule out the presence of beta hemolytic streptococcal infections.

FACTORS AFFECTING THE LENGTH OF THE LATENT PHASE OF LABOR

Cervical Dilatation

The cervical dilatation at time of admission most accurately predicts the remaining length of the labor.[3,4] Averaged for all patients, the latent phase of labor will be 9 hours 27 minutes, if first seen at less than 2 cm dilatation. Latent phase will last 7 hours 46 minutes if the patient is admitted at 2 to 3 cm dilatation. Beyond 3 cm of cervical dilatation the average length of latent phase would be 5 hours 22 minutes (see Table 5.2).

In a multivariate analysis of the known factors associated with a prediction of labor length, cervical dilatation was the most important variable when compared with parity, station, and status of the membranes.[3]

Pelvic Station of Vertex

Descent of the vertex often takes place late in the active phase and continues during the second stage of labor. Many multipara will not display vertex descent until full cervical dilatation takes place. Although most clinicians anticipate a more rapid labor progression when a vertex is low in station (+2+3), statistically, at onset of labor, station shows little effect on the length of latent phase.[3]

Parity

Parity has little observed effect on length of latent phase. It accounted for about 1% of the length of latent phase in a statistical study attempting to define importance of parity, dilatation, and station on labor length.[3] Most factors relating to latent phase labor length were unknown. This is in contrast to the second stage of labor, when parity has a more obvious effect.

Maternal Age

Latent phase of labor is not altered (or lengthened) by maternal age. During labor, in the absence of maternal or fetal pathology, increased worry by the clinician because of factors such as maternal age, statements such as, "This is a very important baby," or because of a history of infertility, are inappropriate and should not influence clinical decisions. For the fetus, who will make only one trip through the pelvis, that one trip is very important. There is little data to suggest that maternal age (without observed pathology such as hypertension) should increase fetal risk or foreshadow a more difficult labor. Similarly, infertility, once overcome, is not a labor management problem.

Rupture of Membranes During Latent Phase

The Cleveland Metropolitan General Hospital review of spontaneous and artificial rupture of membranes confirmed Friedman's earlier studies.[6,8] There was little effect of membrane rupture on labor length. The point to be made is that if it takes sophisticated statistical manipulations on large populations to show small effects, this information, although statistically correct, will not help the clinician's management choices in any individual case.

GUIDELINES FOR ARTIFICIAL RUPTURE OF THE MEMBRANES

If it is accepted that in the average patient membrane rupture does not contribute to the length of labor, when should membranes be ruptured?

1. Routine rupture of membranes is not indicated when labor is progressing satisfactorily. It adds little to rapidity of cervical dilatation.
2. Artificial rupture of membranes (AROM) should be considered if labor is *not* progressing satisfactorily. Perhaps this will change the course of labor. This is not in conflict with the previous statement. In normal labors AROM makes little contribution to rate of cervical change. In slow or prolonged labor the data has not been obtained and a helpful effect is possible. Clinical experience suggests it may be helpful.

   Note that the dilatation effect after membrane rupture is not immediate and may take time. Often, immediately following AROM a small regression in cervical dilatation may take place before the vertex becomes well applied to the cervix.
3. Rupture of membranes may be performed if fetal distress is suspected. It is helpful to know if meconium is present.
4. Rupture of membranes should be performed if internal fetal monitoring is needed and adequate monitoring information cannot be obtained from an abdominal recording.
5. Rupture of membranes should be considered if uterine size is excessive. Note that too rapid contraction of the uterus after volume release may be associated with placental deprivation.

LATENT PHASE LABOR MANAGEMENT

EXAMPLE OF OPTIONS TO ADMITTING PATIENT AND ACTIVELY INTERVENING

A nulliparous patient is seen at term in the labor admitting area. She is experiencing mild contractions every 7 minutes. The cervix is 3 cm dilated, 75% effaced, and the vertex is at S-1. The patient has a normal antenatal history and external fetal heart rate monitoring is unremarkable. It is the admitting physician's opinion that the patient is probably early in latent phase labor. As this is the first patient contact, no progress in cervical dilatation has as yet been observed.

Option 1

Send patient home.

Her labor will be short when she returns. This must be acceptable to the patient.

Option 2

Admit patient and observe.

This decision is often motivated by the patient's apprehension and the distance between her residence and the hospital.

Option 3

Admit patient and induce or augment labor with oxytocin.

This decision is motivated by a clinical judgment that the patient is inducible. Most clinicians would choose this option because at 3 cm and 75% effacement good progress may be anticipated.

Option 4

Rupture membranes and await dilatation or use oxytocin.

This decision is sometimes acceptable, however, once membranes are ruptured there is a commitment to completing labor and maintaining monitoring. If the rupture of membranes has, at best, a small effect on labor length, why rupture the membranes to augment labor? If oxytocin is used and the information obtained by external monitoring is acceptable, routine membrane rupture is not mandatory. You can always turn off the oxytocin if, despite the observed initial cervical dilatation, no progress occurred.

EXAMPLE OF NOT ACTIVELY INTERVENING IN POSSIBLE LATENT PHASE LABOR

A term multipara with vertex at S-3, cervix long posterior and one fingertip dilated, stated she was experiencing contractions every 7 minutes for 24 hours. The fetal heart monitoring taken in the screening area for 30 minutes was normal. Occasional contractions, each 7 to 10 minutes, were seen.

Option 1

Send patient home.

This is fine if acceptable to the patient. If she and her spouse have been up for the past 24 hours counting contractions, she may need more support.

Option 2

Admit patient and use sedation.

This is acceptable if the decision is to rest this patient and use analgesia for pain. Morphine works well in the presence of pain and with a term size fetus. In contrast, use minimal medication in a low-birth-weight fetus. If sleep medication is used when the patient has pain, it may have less effect on this patient. If pain is present use an analgesic.

Option 3

Stimulate patient with oxytocin.

In this case, try to avoid this option. The long cervix foreshadows a long latent phase labor. At the extreme, it may take another 24 hours to reach active phase labor. In this group of patients some will undergo cesareans before they have an adequate trial of labor because of the prolonged length of latent phase. These patients may become difficult management problems.

Option 4

Rupture membranes and stimulate.

This plan is unacceptable for the same reasons expressed in Option 3. Why look for trouble? Later it may be found that no cervical dilation has occurred (or dilatation has not occurred at an acceptable rate). Eight or 10 hours will have passed and pressure to terminate labor will be present.

Although patients at term will often respond to oxytocin use or to membrane rupture when they do not feel inducible, the process is often lengthy and unpredictable. If there are medical indications for this management plan, such as post dates or toxemia, the term "elective" is replaced and we would proceed with the intervention. In the normal patient there is no urgency.

SIX INTERVENTIONS FOR PATIENT MANAGEMENT IN LATENT PHASE

Just as writing an order in the chart or the use of a scalpel is recognized as an intervention, there are six choices for patient care in latent phase labor and all six should be considered before a single intervention is used.

Patience

If the average length of latent phase is understood and the knowledge that a 20-hour latent phase labor is not rare, patience is a most important management tool. A long latent phase does not predict dystocia or fetal distress or infant morbidity. It only foreshadows a tired family and a tired doctor.

Sedation and Analgesia

Subcutaneous morphine doses of 4 mg to as much as 15 mg (dictated by patient size) will allow the patient to rest. Meperidine or other narcotics are also appropriate analgesic alternatives. Prefer the narcotic when pain is present and rest is needed. Rarely use barbiturates for these patients. Following narcotic analgesia, expect a 3- to 4-hour delay in cervical dilatation before progress occurs. In latent phase, the normal slow cervical dilatation may be prolonged further by medications. Avoid routine medication use in latent labor.

A word of caution about morphine use. Do not use it for the normal laboring patient who needs some analgesia. In those cases use meperidine, generally in a 50-mg intravenous route. Use morphine only in a problem situation when the patient needs rest and the fetus is normal.

Regional Anesthesia (Epidural Anesthesia)

Regional anesthesia is frequently used in active labor. However, in latent phase labor an epidural block should be limited to the unusually fearful patient or to the unusually painful labor. It is not unusual that after the epidural block, the physician will have to wait until the anesthetic wears off, or oxytocin may have to be instituted to augment labor.

Oxytocin Augmentation

A common intervention in latent phase labor, oxytocin is used to shorten a long latent phase. If the latent phase is proceeding slowly (eg, 1- to 2-cm dilatation has occurred following several hours of observation) and the nursing personnel are available to monitor the oxytocin infusion, institute oxytocin. A response to oxytocin should be rapid. Following oxytocin use, contractions should begin within minutes and dilatation generally begins within the hour, in contrast to analgesic medication use which usually has a more protracted onset effect on cervical dilatation.

Artificial Rupture of Membrane (AROM)

Despite the fact that statistical analysis has revealed that AROM contributed little to progress in cervical dilation, it is a treatment option. Although engagement may not be present, the vertex should be within the pelvis. Before rupturing the membranes attempt to determine whether the presenting part will descend and be firmly pressed against the cervix. This clinical estimate is accomplished by thinking about what may happen *before* membranes are ruptured. At times, with a high vertex or a large vertex, you can anticipate slow descent. Pressure on the fundus during a vaginal examination may allow you to anticipate descent of the vertex.

If the membranes are ruptured and the vertex does not become well applied to the cervix, there is no dilating wedge and the cervix will not dilate. This is another reason for unfortunate latent phase cesareans. Shortly after membrane rupture, there may be actual regression in cervical dilatation.

It is not clear why, in some cases following AROM, dilatation is rapid and in others no effect may be seen. If the dilating membrane wedge is removed and the vertex does not easily move against the cervix, it may be necessary to wait until molding, flexion, and descent occur before further dilatation takes place.

Patient Position

Another treatment option is to change patient positions. Allow patients to sit or lie in more comfortable positions. Ambulate the patient when possible. In the absence of fetal distress and even in the presence of ruptured membranes (with a head well fit into the pelvis), try to increase patient comfort and do not limit activity. It is not easy for a patient to lay flat on her back (or side) for hours waiting for progress. A lounge area properly monitored by the obstetrical staff is appropriate for many patients.

If membranes are ruptured and the patient leaves the bed, monitoring by auscultation or doptone should continue. Although guidelines for auscultation during latent phase suggest 30 minutes monitoring is acceptable, the choice may be to monitor more frequently during ambulation.

The etiologies for a prolonged latent phase are not known. The six latent phase labor treatments are derived from clinical experience. Many physicians agree that latent phase labor sedation is overused, but at times sedation may be useful during labor.

Use of conduction anesthesia in latent phase labor can be argued. The literature varies in describing outcomes. There is a place for a conduction anesthetic during latent phase. The preference is to use oxytocin more frequently in latent phase and to avoid the epidural block analgesia.

False labor is a management problem. It is wise to keep the early laboring patient out of the labor room when possible. Clinical judgment and use of all choices is encouraged.

CESAREANS AND THE LATENT PHASE OF LABOR

In a study of 2,845 uncomplicated labors (ie, no maternal or fetal emergencies) at Cleveland Metropolitan General Hospital,[3,4] 18 labors (.006%) ended in cesareans before the end of the latent phase of labor. It was clinical policy that no clinician, regardless of experience, was able to predict "dystocia" or "CPD" without a trial of labor. The need for an adequate trial of labor will often be restated in this text. There is no data to suggest that a trial of labor in the vertex presentation is harmful to the fetus, or conversely, that the fetus is healthier if born without labor.

A chart review by a peer group should evaluate decisions. The reason for the review is that patterns of patient care may identify poor obstetrical practices. The decisions noted below should rarely take place.

THE NEED FOR A HOSPITAL POLICY

1. Cesareans are frequently performed during latent labor because of a diagnosis of dystocia.
2. Cesarean without labor takes place because an obstetrician has made the clinical diagnosis that the fetus will not fit through the pelvis.
3. A trial induction is not carried out, or carried out without observed dilatation of the cervix into the active phase prior to terminating.

The key word applied in statements 1, 2, and 3 above is *rarely.* There may be individual decisions based on estimates of excessive size of the fetus (>4500 g) or unique maternal problems.

SUMMARY

1. Latent phase labor begins with the onset of uterine contractions as described by the mother, and progression of cervical dilatation observed by the clinician.
2. Latent phase labor ends and active phase labor begins when cervical dilation rates are 1.2 cm/h for the primipara and 1.5 cm/h for the multipara.
3. At 5 cm of cervical dilatation, no matter how slow the cervical dilatation rate is, a latent phase of labor has ended and active phase is defined.
4. Cervical dilatation at time of admission most accurately predicts length of labor.
5. Artificial rupture of membranes contributes little to normal progress in labor and should not be used as a routine management plan. It should be reserved for labors in which problems of the fetus, or of progress, may be present.
6. Six acceptable management guidelines for latent phase labor are:

a. Patience
b. Sedation or analgesia
c. Regional anesthesia
d. Oxytocin augmentation
e. Artificial rupture of membrane
f. Ambulation and position changes

7. Cesareans performed in latent phase should rarely relate to labor abnormalities and be performed for urgent maternal or fetal indications.

REFERENCES

1. Cohen W, Friedman E: Management of Labor, vol 2. Baltimore, University Park Press, 1983, p 12.
2. O'Driscoll K, Meager D: Management of Labour, vol 5. London, Philadelphia, Toronto, WB Saunders, 1980, p 25.
3. Peisner D, Rosen MG: The latent phase of labor in normal patients: a reassessment. Obstet Gynecol 1985;66:644–648.
4. Peisner D, Rosen MG: Transition from latent to active labor. Obstet Gynecol 1986;68:448–451.
5. Hendricks CH, Brenner WE, Draus G: Normal cervical dilatation pattern in late pregnancy and labor. Am J Obstet Gynecol 1970;106:1065–1082.
6. Friedman EA, Sachtleben MR: Amniotomy and the course of labor. Obstet Gynecol 1963;22:755–770.
7. Intrapartum fetal distress, in: Antenatal Diagnosis, publication 79-1973. Bethesda, MD, National Institutes of Health, 1979, pp 67–68.
8. Rosen MG, Peisner DB: Effect of amniotic membrane rupture on length of labor. Obstet Gynecol 1987;70:604–605.

Chapter 6

Treatment of Latent Phase Labor Abnormalities

OVERVIEW

Although all the labor pattern problems faced by the clinician cannot be completely replicated by clinical examples described in a textbook, diagnostic and management routines are presented in this chapter, along with examples of patient care patterns. A series of questions are posed which should be answered in the written note in the patient's chart. The information is not new to the clinician. Rather, this is a formalized routine or process which will allow for orderly clinical judgment and improved patient care.

OBJECTIVES

At the conclusion of this chapter, the clinician should be able to:

1. Diagnose abnormalities of patients in latent phase labor
2. Describe therapeutic interventions during latent phase labor
3. Understand that treatment options may incorporate several correct treatments for the same patient
4. Conduct an adequate trial of labor designed to avoid unnecessary commitment to end labor in the latent phase (in the absence of fetal or maternal risk)

SIX DIAGNOSTIC ROUTINES FOR LATENT PHASE LABOR

1. Define the parts of latent phase labor
   a. Onset
   b. Interval
   c. End
2. Describe the antenatal history of the patient
3. Evaluate the carrier
4. Evaluate the passenger
5. Evaluate the forces
6. Evaluate the labor history

SIX THERAPEUTIC INTERVENTIONS FOR LATENT PHASE LABOR

What treatments are available for latent phase labor? The available choices include:

1. Patience (time is a treatment)
2. Ambulation
3. Sedation or analgesia (nonregional)
4. Epidural block
5. Stimulation with oxytocin
6. Rupture of membranes

THE SIX DIAGNOSTIC ROUTINES IN DETAIL AND WITH EXAMPLES

Define the Latent Phase

Latent phase labor begins with the onset of maternal contractions until observed cervical dilation takes place, at a rate of 1.2 cm in the primipara and 1.5 cm in the multipara. As noted in Chapter 3, if there is any doubt about the rate of cervical dilatation, at 5 cm the patient is in the active phase of labor. The normal duration of latent labor may be 20 hours in the nullipara and 12 hours in the multipara.

For descriptive purposes, latent phase is divided into three parts: onset, interval, and end of latent phase.

Onset of Latent Phase

This diagnosis is often difficult to make. Extrapolate back to contraction onset in order to time latent phase labor onset. Without observed dilatation it cannot be stated with certainty that the patient is in labor. In the chart note state, after your initial examination, that the patient may be at the onset of latent phase labor.

EXAMPLE OF PRELABOR CERVICAL DILATATION

In the office examination, a nulliparous patient at 41 weeks of gestation was found to have 2–3 cm of cervical dilatation with 80% effacement.

Comment

This cervical dilatation may have been present for the past week. The key words are *observed* active dilatation, and this has not been confirmed. In this example, choose patient treatment not on the belief that the patient is in labor but rather on the basis of the gestational length of 41 weeks. A patient at 41 weeks of gestation with an inducible cervix should be considered appropriate for induction. In contrast, had the same findings been present at 34 weeks of gestation, the patient should have been sent home and encouraged to avoid activity for the next several weeks.

Interval of Latent Phase

You have *observed* that dilatation has taken place. The more rapid rate of dilatation has not exceeded 1.2 cm/h (nullipara) or 1.5 cm/h (multipara). If 5 cm of cervical dilatation has been reached, no matter how long latent phase has been present, treat the patient as if she is in active phase. If rate of dilatation defines active phase, the rate of dilatation may turn into the active phase of labor at 3 or 4 cm if rapid dilation takes place. If progress during this interval phase is slow, interventions are appropriate. A long interval portion of latent phase labor foreshadows a tired patient when active phase labor progresses.

End of Latent Phase

At least two vaginal examinations have been performed confirming that the active phase dilatation rate is not present, or 5 cm dilation has not been reached. The reason for including this "end" as a segment of latent phase is that if there is uncertainty, the patient should be treated as if in the active phase and intervention should be used if progress is prolonged. Generally intervene more rapidly in latent phase labor to stimulate cervical dilatation.

Describe the Antenatal History of the Patient

In the chart note describe preexisting risks that may modify clinical judgment for the carrier, the passenger, and the passageway or birth canal.

Evaluate the Carrier

Review any maternal risk based on the mother's physical size, clinical pelvimetry, and behavioral problems. Record important risks in the chart note.

EXAMPLE OF A CARRIER RISK

A 250-lb, 5-foot-tall primigravid patient is seen in the admitting area. The cervix is 3 cm dilated, 60% effaced, and the vertex is floating above the pelvic brim. Fetal size, although difficult to estimate, is judged to be above 8 lb.

Comment

This clinical picture should suggest the possibility of a problem in pelvic capacity —either bone or soft tissue risks. Labor should be allowed to progress in order to test the pelvis. In most cases these patients, although at risk for maternal–fetal disproportion, deliver vaginally. The outcome of this individual labor cannot be predicted with certainty. Obese patients or patients with excessive weight gain have larger babies. The chart note should describe maternal size as well as the fetal position and size. Obtain ultrasonography to predict fetal size more accurately.

Evaluate the Passenger

Review the evidence for fetal position and size. Look at the maternal abdomen first. Palpate the abdomen. Use Leopold's maneuvers even before using the ultrasound machine, although ultrasonography provides useful information. At the extremes of fetal size (low and high birth weight) the ultrasound measurements have much larger margins of errors.

EXAMPLE OF A PASSENGER PROBLEM

In a multipara with a family history of diabetes and a history of previous vaginal births of 8- and 9-lb neonates, the fetal size on examination was felt to be over 8 lb. The fetal vertex was overlying the pubic symphysis. The cervix was 2 cm dilated. Maternal diabetes was in good control.

Comment

The fetal size should, if possible, be confirmed with ultrasonography—to rule out excessive fetal size—before considering active intervention. Some clinicians suggest that a 4500-g-fetal-size estimate warrants an automatic cesarean. This arbitrary definition is an opinion and not universally accepted. Assess the entire clinical picture including the carrier, the passageway, and the labor.

Individualize the patient's treatment. Aggressive interventions such as oxytocin use are discouraged in these situations. In contrast, in the presence of good progress, such as seen with the vertex descending into pelvis, allow a labor trial.

Ultrasound estimates of fetal size in the very low- and very high-birth-weight ranges have the greatest margins of error. As noted, if labor proceeded spontaneously and the vertex descends in a normal manner, consider vaginal birth. Most clinicians would not use oxytocin nor midforceps later in labor. If vaginal birth is to occur, it will happen on its own. Unexpected shoulder dystocia is increased in the greater than 4500-g fetal group. However, there is room for clinical judgment in the presence of a large fetus.

Evaluate the Forces of Labor

Describe the contraction pattern along with the observed cervical dilatation. Is this effective?

EXAMPLE OF A POSSIBLE CONTRACTION PROBLEM

In a normal term multipara, painful contractions each 4 minutes were observed for 3 hours without any change in cervical dilation. The cervix remained 2 cm dilated and 70% effaced. The vertex was floating and the fetus was estimated to be about 7 lb.

Comment

Latent phase labor onset has not been confirmed despite the presence of contractions. Intervention can be considered.

Treatment with oxytocin is suggested in this example. A second acceptable choice would be to rest the patient with 7 to 12 mg of morphine sulfate given subcutaneously. Morphine rather than a sedative is preferred because painful contractions will not easily be alleviated with a sedative.

Rupturing the membranes at this time would commit the clinician to delivery and it is not certain that the patient is in labor. The forces, or uterine contractions, although painful, have not been effective.

Evaluate the Labor History

Is this patient in labor? Is progress defined? A major problem in latent labor management is ruling out false labor. Once false labor is ruled out, the options include inducing the false labor patient (based on findings), augmenting poor progress in the interval portion of latent phase, or doing nothing and allowing the patient to go home.

EXAMPLE OF EARLY INTERVENTION IN LATENT PHASE LABOR

A multiparous patient was observed to dilate from 1 to 3 cm during the first 3 hours in the labor room. For the next 3 hours there was no progress in cervical dilatation.

Comment

Because dilatation of the cervix has been observed, this patient is in the *interval* portion of latent labor. This latent phase labor is progressing slowly. Consider treatment. Several acceptable treatment choices include: oxytocin, medication, rupture of membranes, or patience.

EXAMPLE OF DIFFICULTY IN DIAGNOSING ONSET OF LATENT PHASE LABOR

A normal multiparous patient at term, with cervix 60% effaced and closed, was observed for 3 hours without cervical dilatation. Contractions were moderate in strength occurring each 5 to 7 minutes. There were no maternal or fetal risks.

Comment

Doubt exists as to whether this labor has begun. Should this patient be induced? There is no medical indication for aggressive management. Therefore, treatment is based on clinical patient evaluation. Judgment between clinicians may differ. This patient may be better served by returning home. It is often better to spend most of latent phase labor at home.

THE SIX THERAPEUTIC INTERVENTIONS FOR LATENT PHASE LABOR

Treatment is usually based on previous evaluations. In order to do this, there should be an attempt to define the latent phase labor, evaluate the maternal and fetal backgrounds, and evaluate the labor history. This leads to therapeutic choices which include the following:

1. Patience
2. Ambulation
3. Sedation or analgesia (nonregional)
4. Epidural block
5. Stimulation with oxytocin
6. Rupture of membranes

Patience

Taking more time is an acceptable treatment for a nonprogressing latent phase labor patient. It is the physician's judgment as to whether patience or a more active form of intervention is needed.

EXAMPLE OF SEVERAL CORRECT THERAPEUTIC CHOICES DURING LATENT PHASE LABOR

A normal nulliparous term patient was seen in the labor screening room with the cervix 1 to 2 cm dilated, 60% effaced, and the vertex at S−3. Irregular but painful contractions every 7 minutes persisted.

Comment

Several choices for treatment in this patient are present. Individualize treatment choices in each situation. If the labor and delivery room is extremely busy at the time of evaluation, this will undoubtedly influence your choice. If the patient has been calling you repeatedly about contractions and false labor, this too will change the choice.

Send the Patient Home

This choice would be acceptable. However, with painful contractions, this may not be possible. Without pain, the low-risk patient belongs at home this early in the latent phase. In this case, in the presence of support persons, waiting in the hospital is acceptable. Remember, this is not the only choice, but it may meet with this patient's needs.

Ambulation

This treatment speaks for itself. It may be useful in any phase of labor but is used most frequently at latent phase labor onset when there is uncertainty that latent labor is present.

Medication

Using medication in latent phase has been both "damned" and "praised." When it is used, the clinician cannot predict what effect it may have on later progress.

Expect a 2- to 4-hour interval of little progress. The choice between whether to stimulate with oxytocin or to be passive (ambulation, patience, medication) is based on the clinician's judgment of the individual patient.

Stimulation with Oxytocin

Oxytocin may give a relatively prompt response documented by progressive cervical effacement and dilatation during the next several hours. If the cervix is poorly effaced, expect some delay until effacement progresses before dilatation takes place. Response by cervical dilatation in latent phase oxytocin augmentation may not be evident for several hours, in contrast to active phase oxytocin use when response should usually be within the hour.

In general, the use of oxytocin is an excellent method to shorten the latent phase and save the patient's energies for later labor when strength will be important. A prolonged latent phase may foreshadow a tired patient during the active phase. To avoid this, intervene earlier in latent phase with stimulation. Monitoring of the fetal heart and frequency of uterine contractions should be performed with electronic devices whenever oxytocin is used. As long as the quality of the information is readable membrane rupture need not be mandated in order to use oxytocin. Failure to make progress in the latent phase of labor, in the absence of membrane rupture, allows the clinician to turn off the oxytocin.

EXAMPLE OF FAILURE TO MAKE PROGRESS FOLLOWING OXYTOCIN USE DURING LATENT PHASE

A normal primigravida at 39 weeks of gestation was seen in the screening area with a vertex presentation, cervix 60% effaced, 2 cm dilated, and 40% effaced. A decision was made to augment or induce, but the clinician could not be certain that the patient was in latent phase labor yet. She was stimulated for 4 hours with oxytocin. Despite regular uterine contractions each 3 minutes, no progress, as defined by cervical dilation, was seen.

Comment

Since the amniotic membranes were not ruptured, there is more flexibility in the next choices. If the fetal monitoring records were normal, the oxytocin stimulation may be stopped and the patient either sedated or sent home when contractions stop. As an alternate treatment, the membranes may be ruptured. However, there is no evidence that latent phase labor *onset* has begun or that AROM will be effective. Expect a long latent phase labor.

Membrane Rupture

This is an active intervention at this time. In the absence of fetal indications it is less acceptable. At 1- to 2-cm dilatation and a high vertex presenting, if membranes are ruptured a long induction can be expected with no withdrawal possible.

EXAMPLE OF LATENT PHASE LABOR INTERVENTION FOR PATIENT NEEDS

A multiparous patient at term was seen in the screening room at 1 to 2 cm of cervical dilation, 60% effaced, station S-3, with a normal fetal and maternal antenatal history. For the previous two nights she had little sleep and was obviously exhausted.

Comment

This patient needs rest. Do not expect a short labor. If pain is the problem, medicate appropriately with a narcotic (meperidine 100 mg or morphine 7–15 mg subcutaneously). If pain is not a problem, perhaps an analgesic such as 200 mg of seconal will suffice to provide sleep. The family should be encouraged to support this approach. The auditory portion of the fetal monitor should be turned down. All low-risk patients need not be monitored. Do not hesitate to remove the abdominal straps and monitoring devices to make the patient more comfortable.

As noted in Chapter 3, AROM is less routinely suggested for use in the management of labor. It does not add to rapid cervical dilatation. There is little evidence to warrant the routine use of this treatment. Use membrane rupture with caution and only perform ROM when committed to completing an already established labor. Most membranes rupture spontaneously in normal labor. The rate of cervical dilation is more rapid following spontaneous rupture of membranes (SROM) rather than AROM.

EXAMPLE OF A MANAGEMENT PROBLEM FOLLOWING AROM DURING LATENT PHASE

A normal nullipara noted 5-minute contractions which began 2 hours earlier. The vertex was X-0, cervix 2 to 3 cm dilated with a normal-sized passenger, and pelvis estimated. Because she was at station 0, it was elected to rupture the membranes. Despite the favorable cervix, dilatation did not occur. The vertex was now poorly applied to a 2- to 3-cm floppy cervix with no observed change during the next 4 hours.

Comment

Nothing but trouble was gained by the membrane rupture. Now the only acceptable choice left for the clinician is to use oxytocin. Eventually in this labor (if the latent phase lasts 12, 18, or 20 hours) there will be some concern about the length of time of the ROM, and worry for infection will be added to the management problems. When AROM works, it is great. When it does not, it is a problem. Since this is often unpredictable, avoid using this treatment early or unnecessarily. The later in labor ROM is performed, the fewer the problems encountered.

Cesarean

As stated previously, the use of the abdominal birth route as a treatment choice in latent labor should be uncommon. In many instances, the selection of this intervention may reflect failure to correctly recognize that latent labor (onset) was not present. Pelvic capacity is not adequately tested by terminating labor with a cesarean during latent phase. In later pregnancies, when discussing the reasons for their cesareans, these patients may recount labors described as 1 or 2 days in length. Yet, the clinician could not be sure they were in labor.

Cesareans are performed in latent phase labor for maternal or fetal indications. These indications may include hemorrhage, infection, fetal distress, and unusual fetal size or presentation.

REVIEWING THE FORMAT FOR ANALYZING AND TREATING LATENT PHASE LABOR

Posing and responding to the following questions will provide a generalized format for a diagnostic process.

Diagnostic Process

1. Is the patient in latent labor? Yes ____ No ____
2. What is the phase of latent labor? Onset ____ Interval ____ End ____
3. Are there background factors or concerns for the carrier, the passenger, the forces? Yes ____ No ____
4. Describe the obstetrical findings including contractions, dilatation of cervix, and station of vertex.
5. Summary statement. The therapeutic choices follow as an outcome of the diagnostic process.

Therapeutic Choices

In your chart notes document the intervention and the time it was instituted.

1. Patience
2. Ambulation
3. Sedation or analgesia
4. Epidural block
5. Stimulation with oxytocin
6. Rupture of membrane

   (Cesareans are rarely appropriate here.)

Diagnostic steps 1 through 5 should be routine parts of patient notes. The therapeutic interventions may take place in varied sequences, depending on clinical progress. *Time* is used to describe the start and finish of an intervention. The program is easily correlated with the graphic labor curves. Either the effect is seen or the effect is not working. Time for effect of the intervention lets the clinician know when to move on. With medication anticipate more time before intervening again, the effects may take hours. Expect more rapid change with oxytocin, usually within the hour.

EXAMPLE OF LATENT PHASE DIAGNOSIS AND TREATMENT

History

On admission, a healthy 28-year-old G3 P2 patient at 41-weeks gestation stated that her contractions had begun 12 hours earlier. At time of admission the contractions were felt to be every 5 to 7 minutes, of moderate intensity, and painful. The patient's membranes were intact. On abdominal examination, the fetus was normal in size with the back on the left and the vertex unengaged. On vaginal examination, the vertex was LOT, S−3, with cervix 1 to 2 cm dilated, posterior, 60% effaced, and soft. The patient's antepartum course was benign and her clinical pelvimetry was unremarkable (see Figure 6.1).

Diagnostic Plan (Chart Note)

We are uncertain that the patient is at the onset of latent labor. Although contractions began 12 hours earlier, there is no labor diagnosis yet. The mother has had a benign antepartum course with normal clinical pelvimetry, the fetus is of normal size and without evidence of risk.

↓ 12 h of contractions pass

Uncertain labor diagnosis exists

Patient is admitted to hospital

Write the Therapeutic Plan in the Chart

The choices include patience, ambulation, medication, epidural block, stimulation with oxytocin, AROM, or cesarean.

Patience

This is the least aggressive mode of therapy. The patient has not been in hospital long enough to make a diagnosis. Many would choose to observe her progress for about 2 hours. Is it possible to send this patient home? Certainly, if this were acceptable to her.

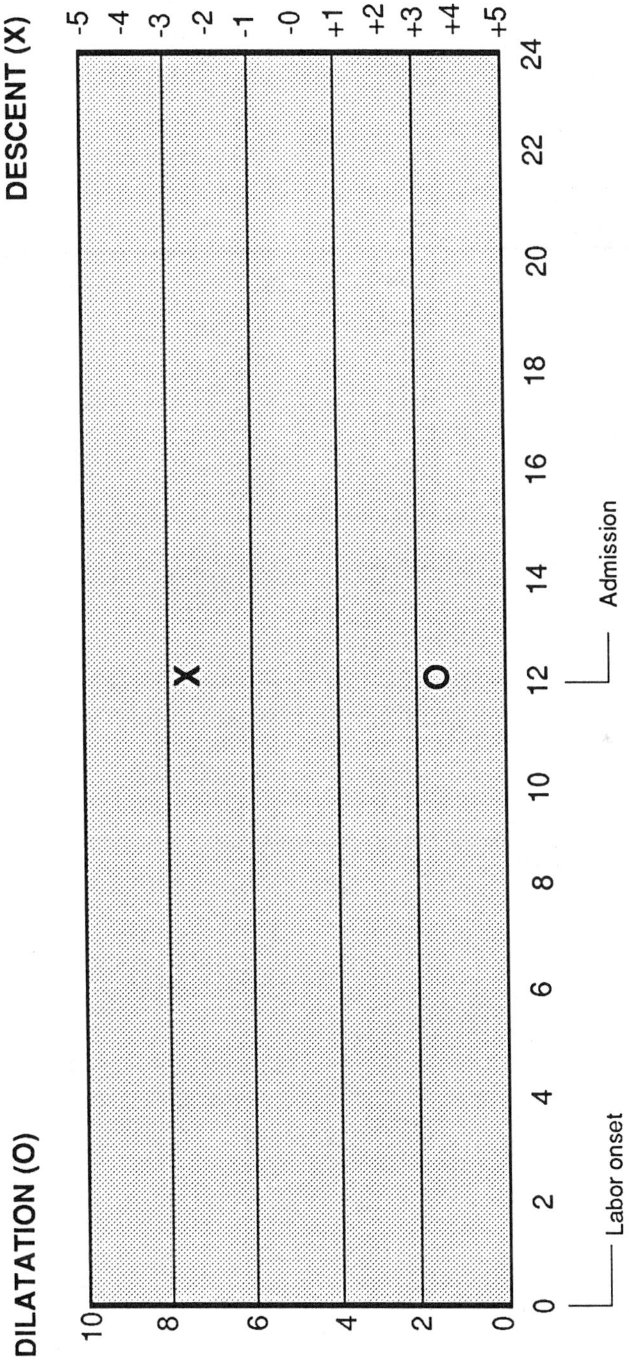
DILATATION (O)
DESCENT (X)
10
8
6
4
2
0
-5
-4
-3
-2
-1
-0
+1
+2
+3
+4
+5
X
O
0
2
4
6
8
10
12
14
16
18
20
22
24
Labor onset
Admission
HOURS IN LABOR

FIGURE 6.1

Ambulation

At the end of a stated time period if nothing changes while in the hospital, plan a new therapy. A time of 1 or 2 hours is more than sufficient for a patient to ambulate.

Medication

This is acceptable if pain is a major problem or if this patient is tired and needs rest. Even if in latent phase labor, expect a delay of at least 2 to 4 hours in cervical response with dilatation. In this patient, pain does not appear to be a problem. The less medication used in latent phase labor, the less confounding factors labor presents.

Epidural Block

This is unacceptable at this time. It is uncertain as to whether or not this patient is in labor. If used in the absence of observed cervical dilation, the need for oxytocin will soon follow. If used, it will need to be continued for many hours.

Oxytocin

This is less acceptable as a long labor is expected (cervix 60%). Why induce in the face of a long labor?

AROM

This is unacceptable at this time. There is no medical reason why this patient must deliver today. Once the membranes are ruptured there is a commitment. If delivery is the choice, oxytocin stimulation provides a more flexible option.

Cesarean

This is not an acceptable intervention. It is not known whether labor will fail because of a small pelvis (see Figure 6.2).

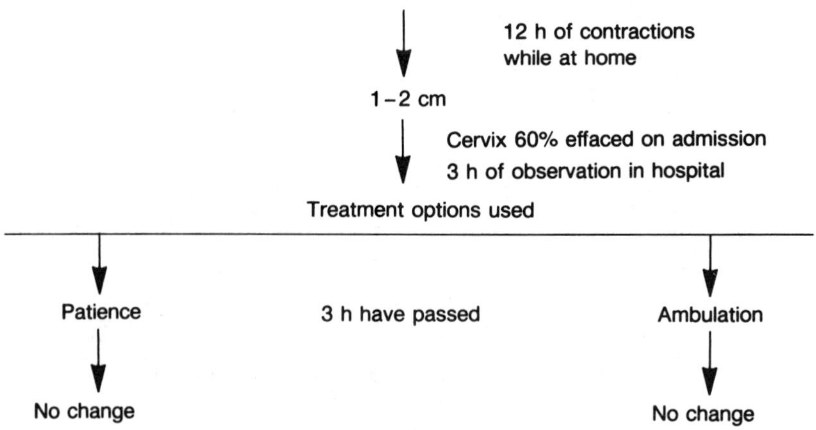

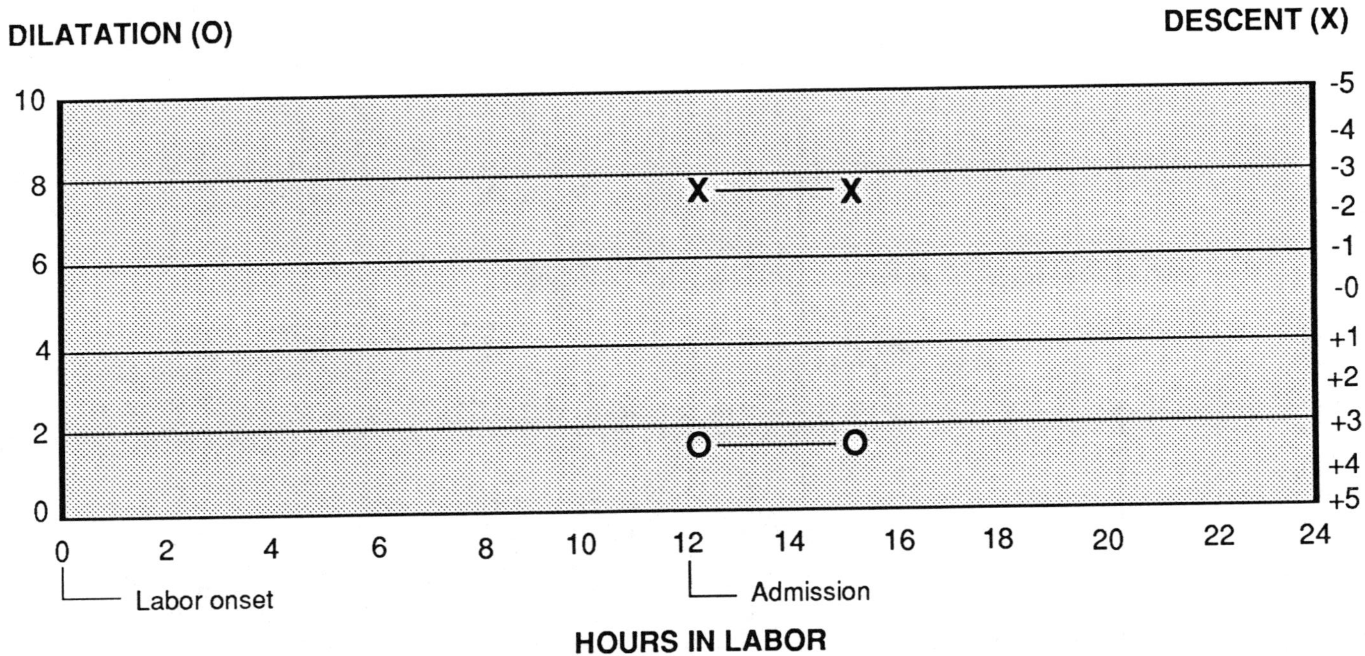
DILATATION (O)
DESCENT (X)
10
8
6
4
2
0
-5
-4
-3
-2
-1
-0
+1
+2
+3
+4
+5
0
2
4
6
8
10
12
14
16
18
20
22
24
Labor onset
Admission
HOURS IN LABOR

FIGURE 6.2

This patient may still be sent home or sedated and observed. If sent home, she may soon return in active labor. Nothing is lost. If sedated, she may wake up in active labor and nothing is lost. If no change occurs after sedation, this patient still may be sent home or labor stimulated with oxytocin. During the observation period the patient should know her physician's opinions—that she may not be in labor—so that she may be sent home.

She was given 100 mg of meperidine intramuscularly for rest (see Figure 6.3).

Meperidine (100 mg)	↓	Cervix 1–2 cm, 60% Labor ?
		4 h pass
Oxytocin considered	↓	Cervix 1–2 cm, 60% Labor ?

It is clear this patient is not in labor. It must be understood that persisting means the patient is being induced. Labor is not being augmented; there is no labor. Dilatation has not occurred; therefore, the diagnosis of labor cannot be made. You may still stop this therapeutic trial after the use of oxytocin. It is a judgment that will vary among physicians.

This example illustrates the very common problem of uncertain labor onset. Treatment must be carefully considered in order to avoid creating new problems. At any point that intervention produced cervical dilatation therapeutic interventions for management of latent phase labor would have continued. When these patients are sent home their management becomes less confusing. In the hospital patient care is confounded because the clinician is more prone to "do something." Usually, cervical change does occur. In the described patient, after 16 to 24 hours of living through the "possibility of labor," the physician's decision-making often offers a commitment to complete the pregnancy. In cases such as this, the frequently occurring problem is false labor. It is important to rule out other confounding problems such as genitourinary infections, placental abruption, gastrointestinal infections, and emotional distress. In the presence of a different mother with fetal or maternal risks, the diagnosis would have altered the therapy and perhaps management would have become more aggressive (ie, hospitalization, induction, or delivery would have been considered).

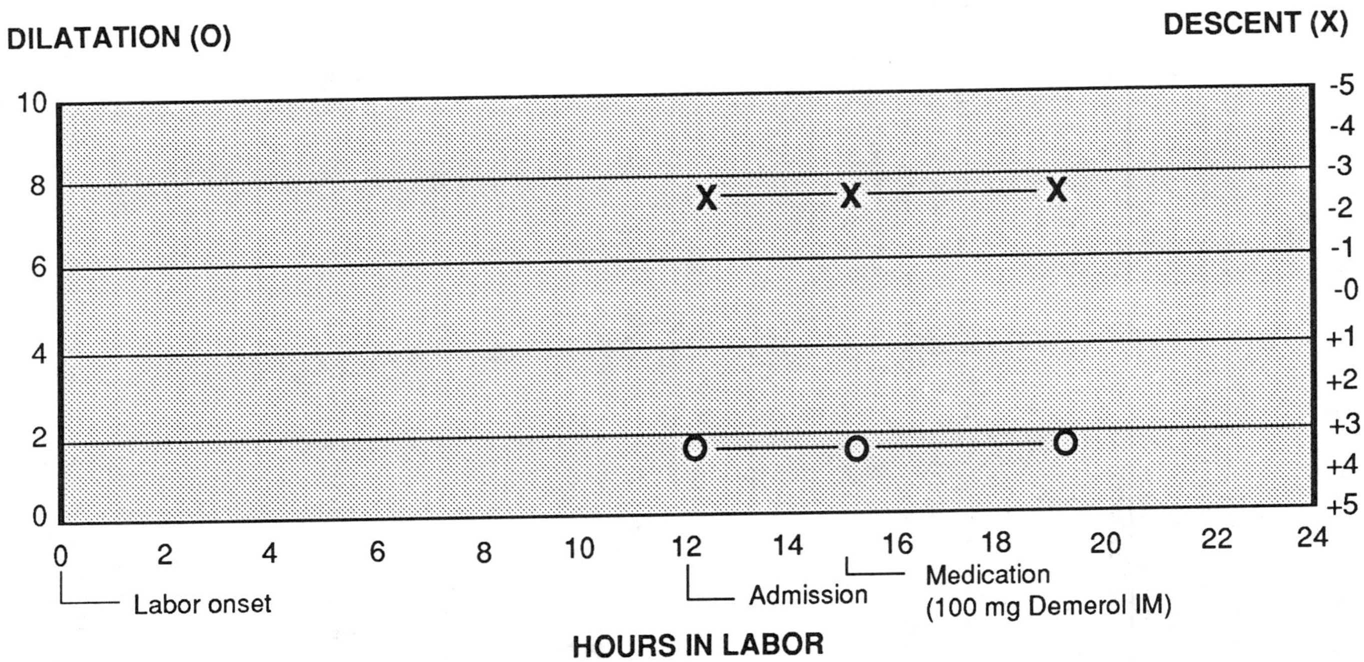
DILATATION (O)
DESCENT (X)
10
8
6
4
2
0
-5
-4
-3
-2
-1
-0
+1
+2
+3
+4
+5
0
2
4
6
8
10
12
14
16
18
20
22
24
Labor onset
Admission
Medication
(100 mg Demerol IM)
HOURS IN LABOR

FIGURE 6.3

EXAMPLE OF LATENT PHASE DIAGNOSIS AND TREATMENT

History

On admission to the labor unit, a 21-year-old multigravida was at 39 weeks of gestation with a normal antepartum history and normal clinical pelvimetry. She was found to be 3 cm dilated, 90% effaced, vertex at station −1 in the LOT, and with irregular uterine contractions, which had begun 3 hours earlier. Her membranes were intact. The patient felt increasing pelvic pressure and back pain (Figure 6.4).

Diagnostic Plan (Chart Note)

Latent labor onset or interval cannot be documented. Cervical dilatation is present but progress has *not yet* been observed. The mother and fetus appear normal. Since the mother is at term with the cervix 3 cm dilated and 90% effaced, she could easily be augmented or induced. Her antepartum course has been normal.

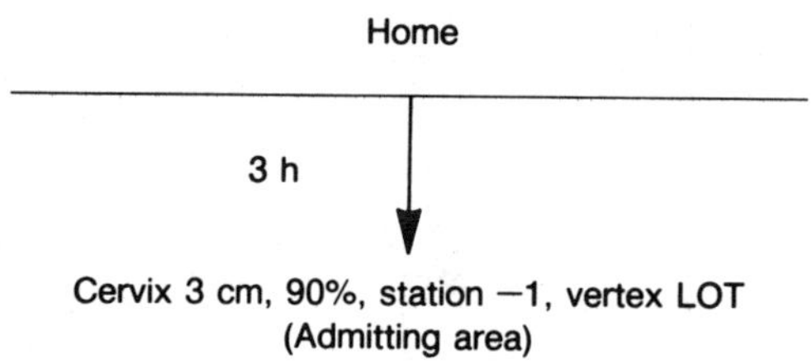

Therapeutic Plan

Patience

This is still possible, but other options may be more acceptable.

Ambulation

This, too, is still possible, but as in the option of patience above, other options may be more acceptable.

Medication

This therapy is not needed. Pain has not been a major symptom.

Epidural or Regional Block

This is not a usual therapeutic pattern in the presence of an easily inducible cervix unless the patient is extremely tired.

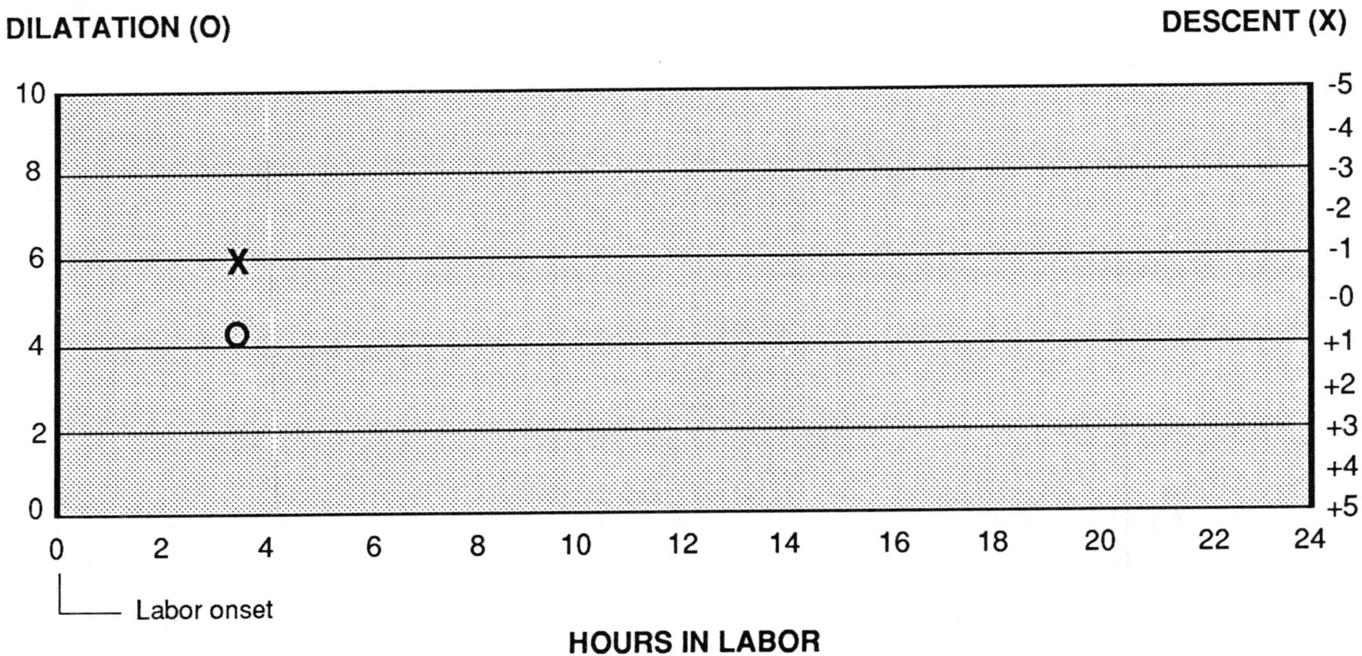
DILATATION (O)
DESCENT (X)
10
8
6
4
2
0
-5
-4
-3
-2
-1
-0
+1
+2
+3
+4
+5
0
2
4
6
8
10
12
14
16
18
20
22
24
Labor onset
HOURS IN LABOR

FIGURE 6.4

Oxytocin

This is the procedure of choice. The oxytocin can be turned off in 4 to 6 hours if nothing happens. At times, even when it seems that the cervix will dilate, it may not. It appears that dilatation will take place in this example.

AROM

This is not a preferred choice. Although AROM may be followed by contractions, the physician is committed to complete the labor. There is no need to be committed to labor completion at this time.

Cesarean

This is not a choice at this stage.

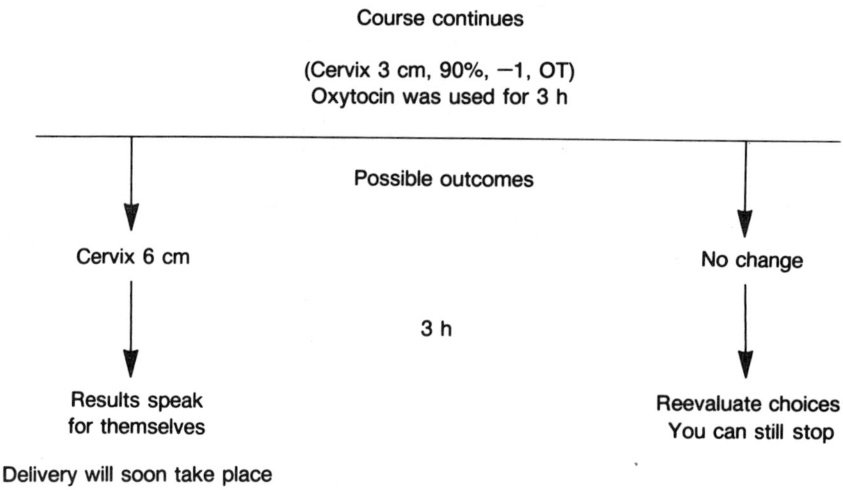

Course

The patient rapidly dilated and entered the active phase of labor. If no change had occurred in 6 hours, the next choice might have been to medicate and rest the patient, then try again the next day, or await onset of spontaneous labor. Membrane rupture commits to an inevitable course, and despite the favorable cervix and the fact that in cases such as this labor will generally follow AROM, it does not always happen. Today, there must be a reason for the increase in the diagnosis of dystocia as an indication for cesareans. Some of this increase in the diagnosis may be due to unnecessary interventions in the term patient who is not in labor.

EXAMPLE OF ACTIVE INTERVENTION IN LATENT PHASE LABOR

History

A 38-year-old multigravida at 42 weeks of gestation, with normal antepartum course, and normal clinical pelvimetry, had a reactive nonstress test 48 hours earlier. She was first seen in the labor screening room with blood pressure 130/80, normal physical and laboratory findings, and an expected normal-size fetus in vertex position. The S−3 vertex was ROT, with cervix 2 cm dilated and 40% effaced. The amniotic membranes were intact. Contractions had been present every 15 minutes for 2 hours.

Diagnostic Plan (Chart Note)

Although labor onset is still uncertain, there is increased risk because of a borderline elevated blood pressure and increased gestational length. Based on these clinical findings, attempt stimulation. The chart note should describe the findings and reasons for therapy.

HOME

2 h ↓

Cervix 2 cm, 40%, ROT (admission findings).

Therapeutic Plan (Chart Note)

Patience

This is neither a likely nor an acceptable therapy. A more aggressive approach at a reasonable hour (or with a rested patient) is indicated for mother and fetus.

Ambulation

This approach is not recommended. The clinical findings have increased the risk factors and the patient should be delivered in an orderly way.

Medication

Pain or exhaustion is not the problem.

Regional Block

Similar to the medication option above, this is not indicated.

Oxytocin

This therapy is the intervention of choice. If progress occurs, you have completed the pregnancy before the risk factors could become more severe. If progress is absent, but the fetus tolerated this prolonged contraction stress test without evidence of distress, the new information will help manage the patient. In the presence of contractions, there does not appear to be fetal risk from deprivation of supply, which is a concern at 42 weeks of gestation and with mild blood pressure elevation.

AROM

There is no need as yet to commit to a delivery today. It would be helpful to document the amount of amniotic fluid on ultrasonography (absence would suggest possible postmature syndrome problems) and perhaps amnioscopy to look for meconium-stained amniotic fluid. The presence of meconium or the absence of amniotic fluid would commit us to completing this labor, which would include AROM if it was felt to be needed.

Cesarean

This is not anticipated and would be a misuse of the information at this time. Even if the induction choice presages a long labor, there is no sign of lack of placental/fetal supply (Figure 6.5).

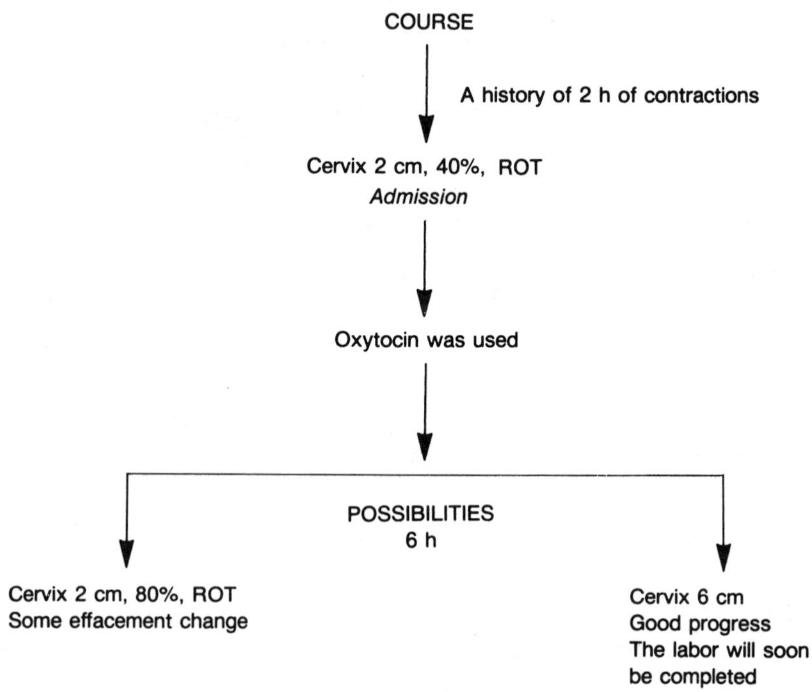

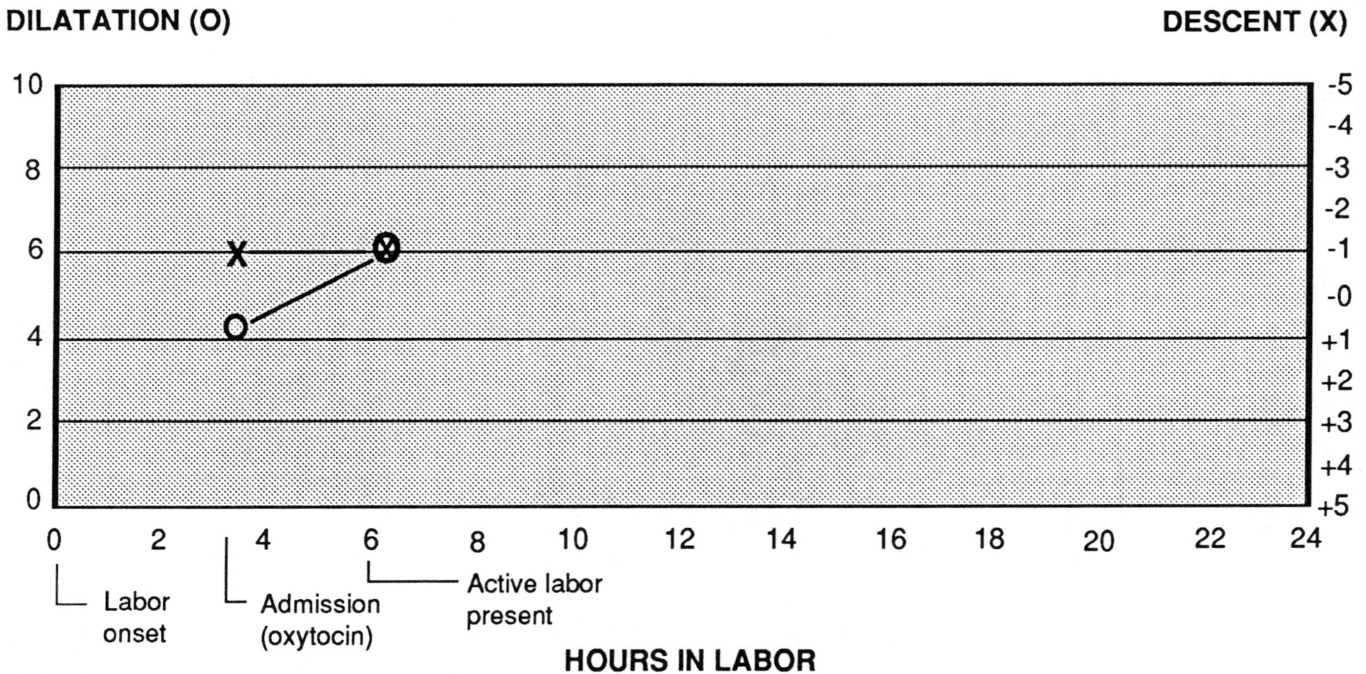
DILATATION (O)
DESCENT (X)
10
8
6
4
2
0
-5
-4
-3
-2
-1
-0
+1
+2
+3
+4
+5
0 2 4 6 8 10 12 14 16 18 20 22 24
Labor onset
Admission (oxytocin)
Active labor present
HOURS IN LABOR

FIGURE 6.5

If, instead of response to oxytocin, no dilatation occurs, the clinician is in a more troublesome position in the treatment process. In the mother's clinical state (no increase in blood pressure), options are still present. Some progress has been made (effacement change from 40% to 80%) and this may be the onset of latent phase labor (no dilatation yet, just effacement).

Therapeutic Choices If No Dilatation Has Occurred

Oxytocin

The clinician may continue as before. This labor may take 20 hours. Be prepared for a long labor, which is acceptable in the absence of fetal distress.

Medication

No reason to use this yet. The patient has not expressed a need for pain relief.

Regional Block

If the patient needs regional block due to behavior (pain, tension, fatigue), use it. In this case it is not an obvious need. This treatment can be used in association with oxytocin to make the patient more comfortable. However, it is more acceptable to use regional block after labor is well established.

AROM

A possible choice, but in view of the cervix, wait unless a change in fetal or maternal conditions warrants a more aggressive approach. For example, if at any time monitoring information was technically poor or confusing with regard to fetal distress, rupture the membranes. As noted on several occasions, in the presence of good quality recordings do not feel ROM and internal monitoring must take place, even if oxytocin is being used.

Cesarean

This is unacceptable in the absence of fetal heart rate abnormalities.

These examples of latent phase labor abnormalities have been presented in terms of diagnostic evaluations and therapeutic plans. The key is *orderly patient care.* Use *all* available information to evaluate the patient. Consider *all* treatment programs. The interventions described encourage *flexibilty of choice* and the use of patient care options which do not compel completion of labor until the decision becomes mandatory based on new patient risks.

SUMMARY

1. When the patient is first seen on hospital admission, the chart note should:

a. Define the latent phase
b. Describe the patient's earlier pregnancy history
c. Evaluate the carrier
d. Evaluate the passenger
e. Evaluate the forces
f. Evaluate the labor history

2. The six clinical treatment choices available during latent phase labor include:

a. Patience
b. Ambulation
c. Sedation or analgesia
d. Epidural block
e. Stimulation with oxytocin
f. Rupture of membranes

3. Therapeutic options may be used in varied orders. If possible, avoid epidural block in early latent phase labor.
4. Avoid interventions such as AROM in early latent phase labor unless there are specific reasons for ending the pregnancy at that time.
5. Cesareans in latent phase labor should only be performed for maternal or fetal risks which are well documented.
6. Cesareans in latent phase labor because of failure to progress should be rare and may indicate the obstetrician's failure to adequately allow an appropriate trial of labor.

Chapter 7

Active Phase and Second Stage of Labor

OVERVIEW

If there is uncertainty as to when latent phase has been completed and active labor has begun, confusion is added to the conduct of labor. The problem for the clinician is to know when active phase of labor has begun, as during active phase labor more rapid interventions are required. Each change in a labor phase sets off a different series of clinical expectations. But even during active phase labor, patience by the clinician and allowing time for labor to progress are primary treatments. In the absence of fetal risk or fetal distress, labor can often go "a little longer" before a decision to end it is reached.

In contrast with the latent phase of labor, dystocia can be diagnosed before the end of active phase. If about 28% of the cesarean birthrate is associated with the diagnosis of dystocia, then better understanding of active phase labor management may lower the cesarean birthrate.[1]

Definitions for durations of latent phase, active phase, and second stage of labor are derived from averaging the lengths of labor of individual patients. It is harder to define the expectations of the birth process taking place during latent and active phase labor than during active and second stages of labor. As an example, in the labor of some patients vertex descent is already present early in labor. For most patients vertex descent is less common during latent phase, more common during active phase, and most common during the second stage of labor. Vertex descent and pelvic capacity are difficult to predict without an adequate trial of the active and second stages of labor.

OBJECTIVES

At the conclusion of this chapter, the clinician should be able to:

1. Define the three parts of active phase labor
2. Complete chart notes to document the patient's course
3. Use graphs for visual descriptions of active labor
4. Understand the relationship of vertex descent to the active phase of labor and to the second stage of labor
5. Understand all the therapeutic interventions for active phase labor
6. Understand the relationship between the end of active phase labor and the onset of the second stage of labor

CERVICAL DILATATION AND ONSET OF THE ACTIVE PHASE

As noted in Chapter 5 at 4 cm of cervical dilatation, about 50% of patients in labor were already dilating at rates greater than 1.2 or 1.5 cm/h, and almost 90% of all patients had reached this rate of dilatation by 5 cm.[2] All patients should be considered to be in active phase labor at 5 cm of cervical dilatation. The change in cervical dilatation rate from the slow latent phase to the rapid active phase is defined as the accelerative portion of active phase labor. A slow accelerative phase may need intervention.

EXAMPLE OF A SLOW ACCELERATION DURING THE ACTIVE PHASE (Figure 7.1)

A primigravida, whose contractions began at 7 PM the previous evening, was 4 cm dilated at 7 AM when first seen by the clinician. At 9 AM the cervix was 4 to 5 cm dilated and in ROT position. At 11 AM she was 5 cm dilated.

Comment

While this is not an arrest, the rate of dilatation is slow. Although the rate of dilatation suggests that this is still latent phase, according to the 5-cm rule the patient is in active labor and should be treated as if in active phase labor, but this is a protraction of the active phase. The slow dilatation of the cervix may need intervention. The chart note should describe whether there are any fetal problems in position, station, or size. Are contractions adequate? Is the mother exhausted or in a great deal of pain? The description in the patient's chart helps to formulate treatment. In order to avoid patient exhaustion act early in treating this labor.

CHARTING ACTIVE PHASE DILATATIONS

The labor graphs used in this text are the Friedman curves.[3] A different charting method is a straight line progression of labor rather than a curve with different slopes of cervical dilatation. The active management protocol of the National Maternity Center states that cervical dilatation rates of 1 cm each hour should be expected. Oxytocin is used for primigravidas if this rate is not reached or maintained.[4] This graphic method is not derived from actual labor experience but is more easily understood.

In contrast, the Friedman graph uses rates of cervical dilatation and descent of the vertex derived from patient measurements, and the plotted curve has several slopes[3] (Figure 7.2). In this text the model Friedman curves for cervical dilatation or vertex descent are not superimposed on the graphs. The idealized dilatation curves are helpful in making a clinical decision; however, too often deviation of a patient's cervical dilatation or descent rate from the classical labor pattern encourages the clinician to end labor. Plot the patient's progress in labor. Visualize whether progress is continuing. Intervene when progress is unacceptable. Deviation from an expected labor curve does not mean medical injury. An elevated patient temperature warrants investigation, diagnosis, and treatment. A slow active phase cervical dilatation rate warrants the same understanding and consideration for treatment. Being aware of the event is important; flexibility of treatment is the art of obstetrics.

THE THREE PARTS OF ACTIVE PHASE LABOR (Figure 7.2)

A–B Accelerative: A slow rate change or transition from latent to active

B–C Maximum slope dilation: A rapid rate change

C–D Decelerative: A slowing in active phase until molding, descent, or rotation takes place and second stage begins

Accelerative Phase

At the transition from latent to active phase labor, the cervical dilatation rate increases. This is seen in Figure 7.2 between points A and B. When there is movement from a slower to a more rapid rate of cervical dilatation, the patient's labor chart reflects this with an abrupt upward change in the slope of the line. This portion of the graph describes the *accelerative phase* of active labor. There may be confusion as to when latent labor ends and active labor begins.

Many patients are in the active phase of labor, as defined by their rate of cervical dilatation, before 4 cm dilatation is reached. These patients may dilate the cervix more rapidly and earlier, but they are not problem cases.[2]

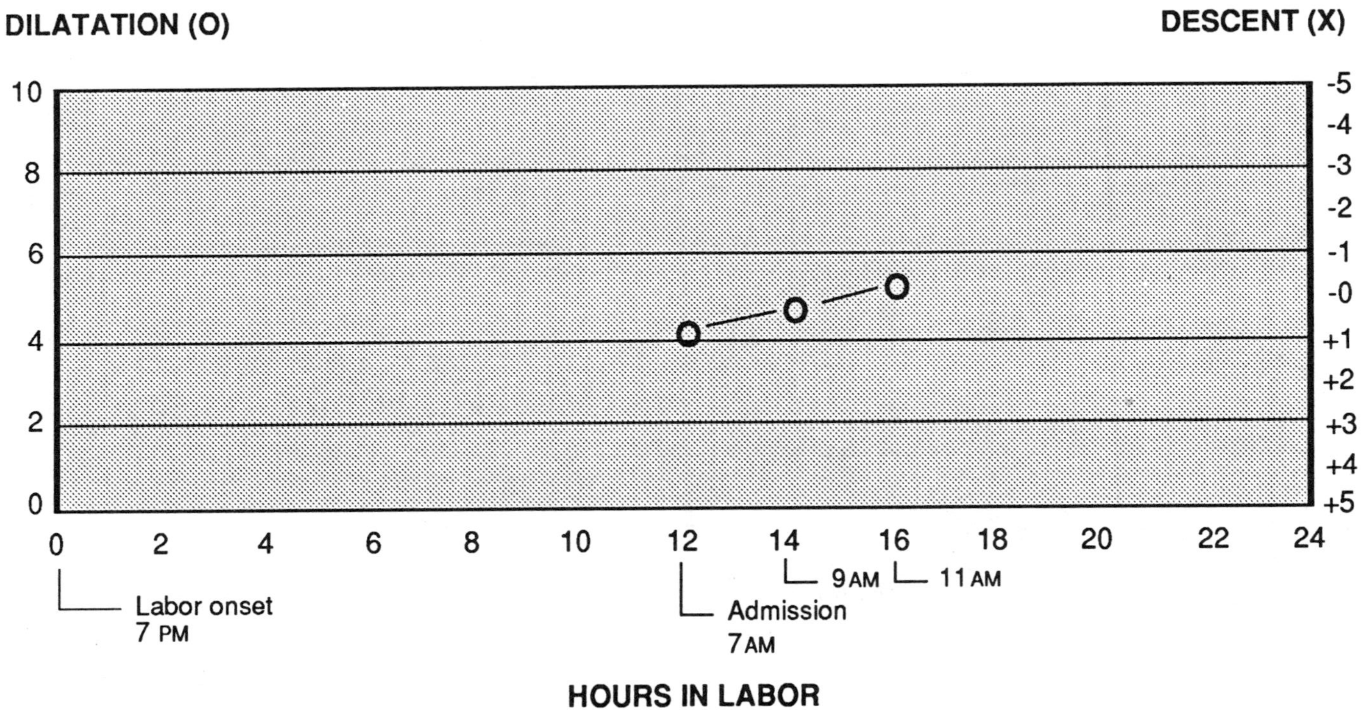
DILATATION (O)
DESCENT (X)
10
8
6
4
2
0
-5
-4
-3
-2
-1
-0
+1
+2
+3
+4
+5
0
2
4
6
8
10
12
14
16
18
20
22
24
Labor onset
7 PM
Admission
7AM
9AM
11AM
HOURS IN LABOR

FIGURE 7.1

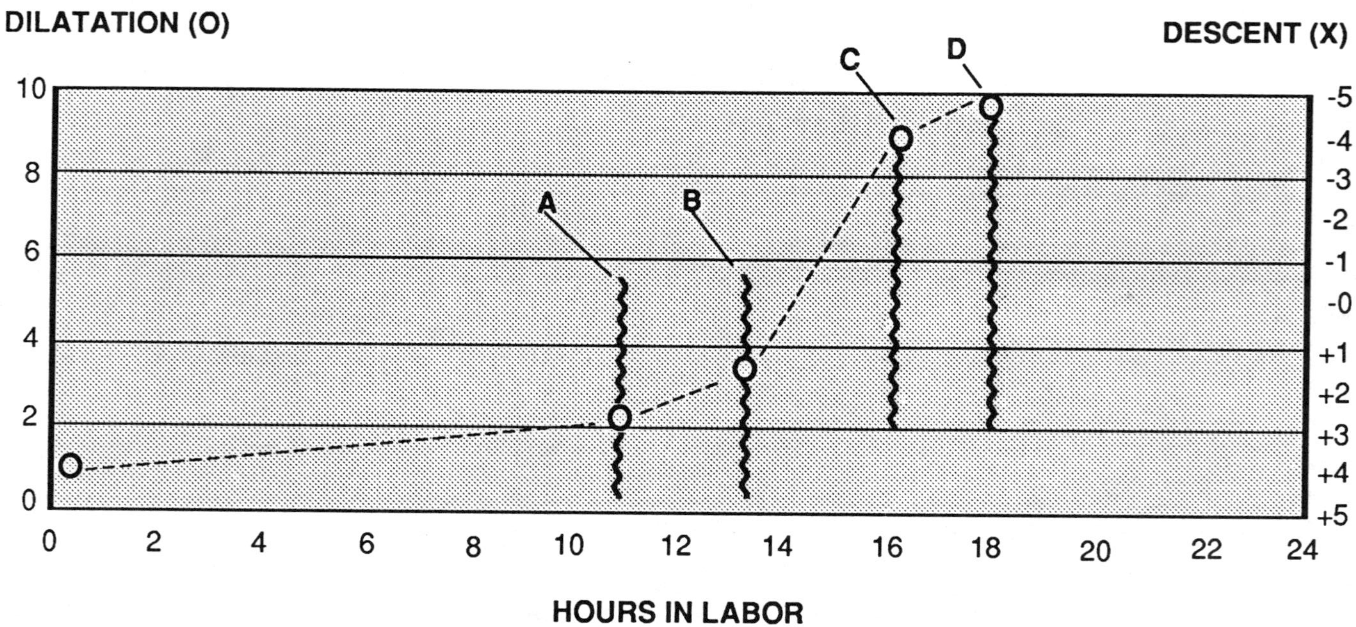
DILATATION (O)
DESCENT (X)
10
8
6
4
2
0
-5
-4
-3
-2
-1
-0
+1
+2
+3
+4
+5
A
B
C
D
0
2
4
6
8
10
12
14
16
18
20
22
24
HOURS IN LABOR

FIGURE 7.2

Maximum Dilatation Phase

Cervical dilation usually continues rapidly throughout most of the active phase. This is seen in Figure 7.2 between points B and C. The more vertical slope defines the *maximum dilatation phase.* The general rate of dilation of the cervix in active phase is 1.2 or 1.5 cm/h, depending on parity (nullipara or multipara). Plot the laboring patient's progress. The clinician's judgment should not be limited by the classic picture of the population's progress. As noted earlier, 1 cm dilatation is an acceptable rate of change each hour. In this range, progress is continuous and there is little reason to intervene. The key word is "continuing" progress. If the patient is not continuing to progress, make a clinical diagnosis of a protraction or an arrest and consider treatment.

Decelerative Phase

The rate of cervical dilatation may slow as it approaches complete dilatation (see Figure 7.2 between points C and D). The presence of a rim of cervix or a lip of cervix often persists longer than expected. Although the existence of the decelerative phase is debated, decelerative phase is present and more often seen in non-occiput-anterior vertex presentations. The occiput posterior or transverse vertex may not reach full dilatation until some descent and some rotation of the vertex occurs. In these positions the disappearance of the remaining cervix takes longer, and the time interval is the decelerative phase. In some patients it is expected that there may be a slowing of cervical dilatation as the vertex begins to descend, rotate, flex, and mold prior to the second stage of labor. The slowing is normal.

PROTRACTIONS AND ARRESTS OF CERVICAL DILATATION

Protractions and arrests in the active phase of labor will be presented again in Chapter 10. Protractions and arrests have been defined by Cohen and Friedman[3] (Table 7.1) and the incidence of the problems has been described by Bottoms et al[5] (Table 7.2) from the Cleveland data. This information is useful and helps to provide terms to describe the labor. It also provides guidelines for determining when labor deviates from the expected course and when interventions should be considered. The recognition of a protraction or an arrest is more easily diagnosed if the labor is graphed (Figure 7.3).

A summary of labor abnormalities at Cleveland Metropolitan General Hospital was derived from a data set of station and dilation recorded in the chart during labor. Table 7.2 reviews the data.

TABLE 7.1 Protractions and Arrests of Cervical Dilatation

	Nulliparas	Multipara (%)
Protracted active-phase dilatation	Maximum slope of dilatation of 1.2 cm/h or less	Maximum slope of 1.5 cm/h or less
Prolonged deceleration phase	Deceleration phase duration of 3h or more	Deceleration phase duration of 1h or more
Secondary arrest of dilatation	Cessation of active-phase progression for 2h or more	

After Friedman.

ASSESSMENT OF DILATION IN THE ACTIVE PHASE

Defining three parts of active phase labor may be helpful in determining patient progress. During active phase labor, a vaginal examination usually should be performed about once each hour. If dilation is not increasing at about 1 cm each hour, reassess the clinical situation.

Progress of less than 1 cm per hour may not be satisfactory. The term "may" is used because it implies judgment for each individual patient. It is best not to set rigid limits for interventions.

When the cervical dilation rate falls to less than 1 cm each hour, the clinician needs to be aware of the rate in order to confirm a labor diagnosis. A judgment can then be made as to whether intervention is what a laboring patient needs. There may not be a need to intervene. In contrast, if three consecutive hourly examinations document an arrest of dilatation, consider the several medical interventions.

TABLE 7.2 Abnormal Labor Patterns[a]

Nullipara (%)		Multipara (%)
>21 h (3.6%)	Prolonged latent phase	>14 h (4.2%)
<1.2 cm/h (25.6%)	Protracted active phase	Dilatation <1.5 cm/h (16.2%)
No change for 2 h (3.6%)	Secondary arrest dilatation	No change for 2 h (6.8%)
Dilatation <1 cm/h (10.4%)	Protracted descent	Dilatation <2 cm/h (4.5%)
No change for 1 h (5.6%)	Arrest descent	No change for ½ h (2.3%)

[a]Incidence at Cleveland Metropolitan Hospital. Modified from Sokol et al.[9]

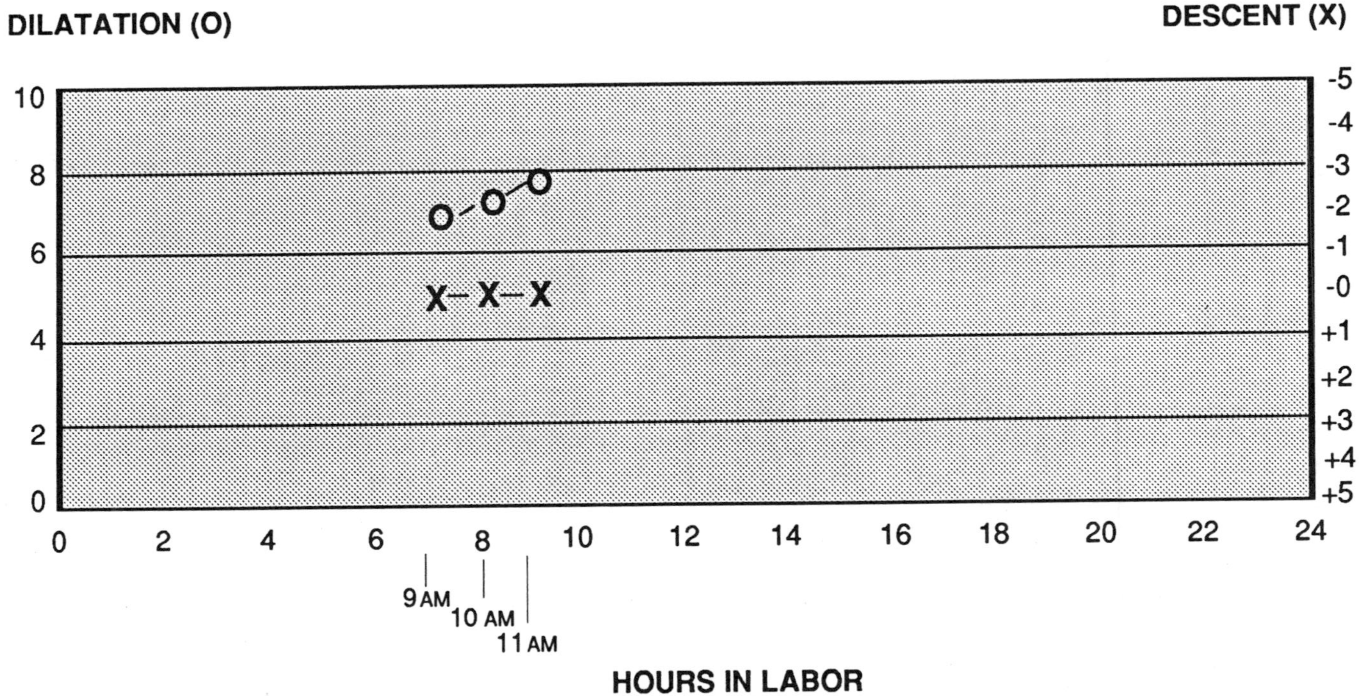
DILATATION (O)
DESCENT (X)
10
8
6
4
2
0
-5
-4
-3
-2
-1
-0
+1
+2
+3
+4
+5
0
2
4
6
8
10
12
14
16
18
20
22
24
9 AM
10 AM
11 AM
HOURS IN LABOR

FIGURE 7.3

EXAMPLE OF PROTRACTION IN THE ACTIVE PHASE (Figure 7.3)

At term, in a normal pregnancy of a P2 G3 mother, the cervix was 7 cm dilated and the vertex was at station 0 in the ROA position at 9 AM. At 10 AM the cervix was 7 to 8 cm dilated and the vertex was S−0. At 11 AM the cervix was 8 cm dilated with no change in station.

Comment

This is not an active phase arrest. According to our expectations, the maximum slope of dilatation should have taken place, but it did not. This active phase of labor is *protracted.* Assess the problem and use clinical judgment to treat this patient based on the patient's needs. Possible interventions at this time could include (1) patience (do nothing), (2) ambulation, (3) augmentation with oxytocin, (4) use of analgesia, (5) regional block, or (6) membrane rupture. Vertex descent is not normally expected at this time.

EXAMPLE OF PROTRACTION IN THE ACTIVE PHASE (Figure 7.4)

A P2 G3 term patient with vertex in the LOP position was found to be 8 cm dilated at 1 PM. At 3 PM she was 9 cm dilated. The vertex position and station were unchanged.

Comment

This case fits the definition of a protraction of the active phase. Consider intervention. Expect slower cervical dilatation with the vertex in posterior or transverse positions, or with a poorly flexed head. The cervix may not retract as rapidly until further descent and rotation take place. Interventions include *no* intervention, ie, patience (a tincture of time is an acceptable intervention), or any of the measures noted in the previous example, including analgesia or oxytocin. Do not consider cesarean because the labor should continue. With an incompletely dilated cervix, forceps should not be considered. The use of vacuum extraction will be discussed in Chapter 12. Be wary of performing vacuum extraction at higher pelvic stations or to the *"almost"* fully dilated cervices.

DESCENT PHASES OF ACTIVE LABOR

Because vertex descent may overlap active phase labor, it is described here as well as in Chapter 8.

Onset

Vertex descent usually begins late in the active phase. In many labors descent may not begin until the cervix is fully dilated. Descent may occur

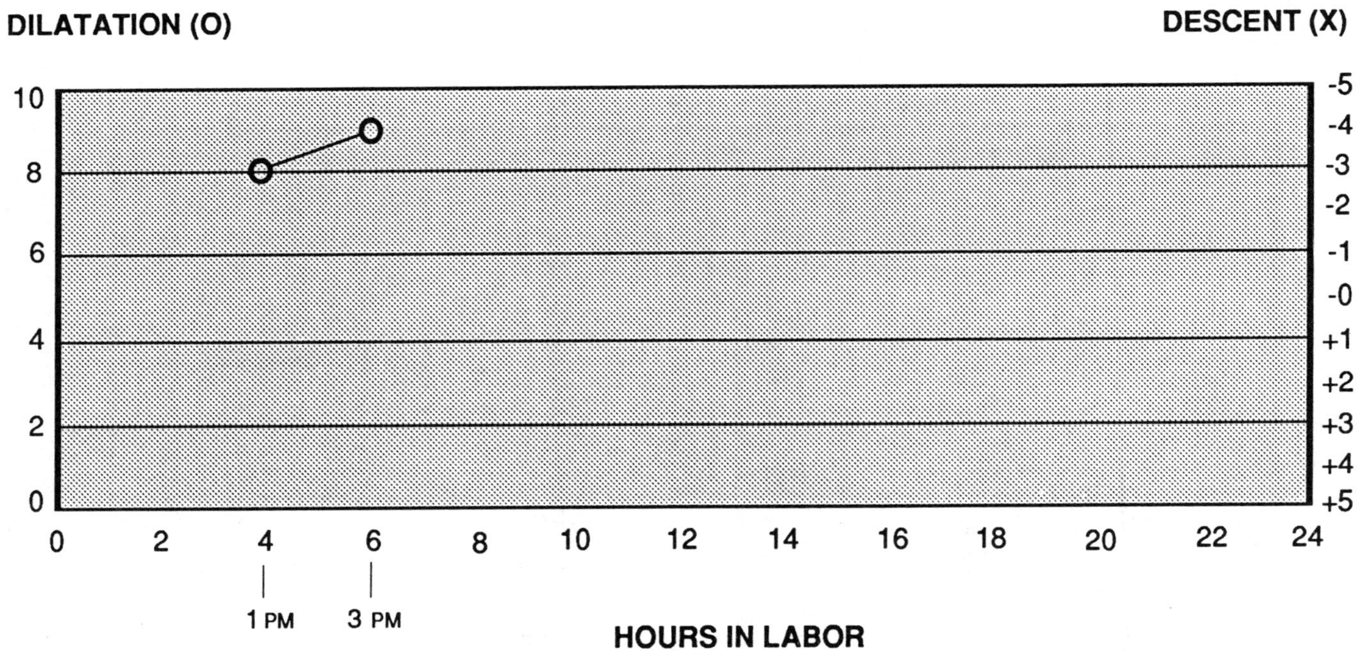
DILATATION (O)
DESCENT (X)
10
8
6
4
2
0
-5
-4
-3
-2
-1
-0
+1
+2
+3
+4
+5
0
2
4
6
8
10
12
14
16
18
20
22
24
1 PM
3 PM
HOURS IN LABOR

FIGURE 7.4

TABLE 7.3 Abnormalities of Descent

	Nullipara	Multipara
Protraction	<1 cm dilatation change/h	<2 cm dilatation change/h
Arrest	No change in dilatation in an h	No change in dilatation in 30 min

After Friedman.

later in the multipara but usually progresses with greater rapidity once it starts. In the nullipara, the vertex is usually at lower stations on admission, but descent occurs more slowly. If, after full dilatation between two vaginal examinations one hour apart descent has not begun or having begun stops, either a protraction or an arrest is defined (Table 7.3).

Arrest

In contrast to cervical dilatation, clinical difficulties in managing vertex descent in the second stage of labor may be more morbid. Rarely should delivery be attempted through an incompletely dilated cervix. A high forceps intervention should not be attempted in today's practice of obstetrics except in the most extreme emergencies. Today, some clinicians use vacuum extraction at less than complete stages of cervical dilatation. The extractor should be applied cautiously.

FACTORS CONFOUNDING EVALUATION OF ACTIVE PHASE DESCENT

Confusion in evaluating descent may be encountered because of caput formation and molding of the vertex. Both formation of caput and vertex molding will take place in the absence of descent, and in performing a vaginal examination the clinician must allow for these fetal changes when estimating change of station. The longer the labor, the easier it is to incorrectly estimate that greater descent has occurred when, in fact, only vertex molding and caput formation have taken place. Be conservative and if in doubt, underestimate the pelvic station of the vertex.

Transverse and occiput posterior positions also confuse estimation of descent. More molding and caput may form and more time will be needed for descent to take place. In occiput posterior position the vertex is usually poorly flexed and the biparietal diameter is farther from the presenting part of the vertex. More errors may be made by the clinician inferring lower station than actually may exist. Over the years, the use of forceps in these situations has decreased and this is to be encouraged. The choice of a difficult forceps after an abnormal second stage should be uncommon.

FOUR FACTORS ALTERING PROGRESS IN ACTIVE PHASE

Parity
Station
Dilatation
Membranes

Clinical management is an art rather than a single pattern of care. Patient care must be individualized. Previous clinical experiences provide the basis for judgment and interventions.

In labor, evaluating the importance of many of the variables affecting cervical dilatation and vertex descent is difficult. Rates for the length of labor are guides. The mother in labor requires individualized assessment.

The beginning clinician prefers a number to be given, or a line to be drawn, beyond which an action should be taken. There is, in fact, a great deal of latitude for patient care during labor. In the absence of fetal distress, there is no rush to complete the labor.

Parity and Its Contribution to Labor Length

We expect nulliparas to progress differently than multiparas during labor. Nulliparas generally have longer latent phases and longer second stages. In contrast, during active phase the numbers 1.2 cm and 1.5 cm/h represent little measurable differences in cervical dilation rates and are difficult to perceive when attempting to estimate cervical dilation during a vaginal examination—a most imprecise measurement.

EXAMPLE OF THE LACK OF MEANING OF THE PRECISE DILATATION RATE

Using the rate of cervical dilatation of 1.2 cm/h for nulliparas and 1.5 cm/h for multiparas, the majority of patients in the two groups will have rates of dilatation between 1 and 2 cm and progress will appear to be the same throughout labor. It is only when hundreds of labors are averaged that the differences become apparent.

EXAMPLE OF THE LACK OF MEANING OF THE PRECISE LENGTH OF ACTIVE LABOR

The length of active phase for the nulliparous patient group is 5 hours. The length of active phase for the multiparous group is 4 hours. Once again the numerical differences are hardly of use. More often the length of the latent and second stages correlate more closely with parity and parity contributes more to labor length.[3]

Vertex Station: A Need To Use the Same Measurements

Use five stations above and below the ischial spines. Some clinicians use three stations of the pelvis, which relates to finger breadths above or below the spine. Today, most clinicians use centimeter divisions (also an estimate) and five pelvic stations (Table 7.4). For simplicity in understanding descriptions of labor, use this terminology.

In Table 7.4, if the presenting part is palpated at or below the ischial spines, the widest part of the vertex presentation may be expected to be within the pelvic inlet. At that point anticipate that vaginal birth should not be obstructed due to bony disproportion between size of the vertex and size of the pelvis. If the vertex is occiput posterior or occiput transverse, the distance between the fetal presenting part and the entrance of the fetal biparietal diameter into the inlet is longer. And although the head may feel engaged, the tip of the presenting part must be palpated at a lower station than 0, or the widest vertex diameter may still be above the inlet.

Consider also caput and molding of the vertex. These factors, when present, contribute to a more conservative estimate of the station of the vertex. It is safer to estimate a vertex higher than it feels to be.

EXAMPLE OF PELVIC STATION AND PREDICTING LABOR LENGTH

A primigravida at station +3 (of five stations) still has significant time before crowning and birth. In contrast, S+3 (of three stations) suggests imminent delivery.

TABLE 7.4 Pelvic Stations

Three Pelvic Stations	Five Pelvic Stations	
−3	−5	Pelvic inlet
−2	−4	
	−3	
−1	−2	
	−1	
0	0	Ischial spines (engagement)
1	1	
	2	
2	3	
	4	
3	5	On the perineum (vertex in view with contraction)

Comment

This may seem insignificant. However, a forceps is a midforceps at S+3 of five stations, and a low or outlet forceps at S+3 of three stations. In the courtroom this is useful information. It is time all concerned use the same definitions; five stations to define the pelvis should become standard. In Chapter 11 forceps will also be defined by pelvic station.

Vertex Station and Its Contribution to Labor Length

Earlier in labor the fetus of the nullipara is usually lower in the pelvis than the fetus of the multipara. In the nullipara, descent to S+5 (the perineum) may occur later in active or second stage and will be slower when compared with the descent in the multipara, in which descent, once started, moves rapidly. Station of the vertex at labor onset contributes little to the length of labor. That is, 1% of the known reasons for length of labor are influenced by station of vertex in the pelvis.[2]

It is important to place station of the vertex in proper perspective for clinical use. A high station for the nullipara or multipara may be associated with a longer labor, although station is not the major predictive factor of labor length. Similarly, a high pelvic station does not allow the clinician to predict labor failure prior to a trial of labor. In an extreme case, if the vertex is out of the pelvis, perhaps even overriding the symphysis pubis, the clinician should be looking for reasons for this fetal position. Is the patient obese? Is the placenta low-lying or a placenta previa? Is the fetus of excessive size or is the vertex abnormal in shape? Is a pelvic kidney present? (Pelvic kidneys may not always obstruct vertex descent.) In the absence of overt pathology, even in the presence of the high vertex, a labor trial is indicated.

Cervical Dilatation and Labor Length

In contrast to station and parity, dilation of the cervix contributes more to the clinician's ability to predict how long the labor will be. About 4% of the known reasons for length of labor are derived from cervical dilatation.[2] In reality, this amount is not really very helpful as most reasons for labor length are not quantifiable. For example, one cannot quantify the effect of maternal contractions, position and flexion of the fetal vertex, or maternal relaxation or position during labor, and predict how these variables influence labor length. Many parts of labor are still not defined scientifically. Estimating and judging are arts that improve with clinical experience.

Amniotic Membranes and Labor Length

Large patient populations and sophisticated statistical analysis are needed to document the very small (1%) known effect of artificial membrane rupture (AROM) on length of labor.[2] With this knowledge in mind, there should be no routine plan to rupture membranes for the individual patient. In some patients AROM will help speed up labor. In others, it may hinder progress. In most cases, artificial membrane rupture is of little help.

EXAMPLE OF DECIDING ON WHETHER TO RUPTURE THE MEMBRANES

At entry into the labor suite, a multipara was found to be a vertex presentation LOT, with cervix 5 cm dilated and at station 0. The amniotic membranes were intact. How should the membranes be managed?

Comment

Some obstetricians routinely rupture membranes at this time. However, when there are no patient problems, there is little to be gained. Why rupture membranes now? If progress is good, there is no need to intervene. Membranes should not be ruptured to routinely visualize amniotic fluid or to insert internal fetal monitors in the absence of fetal or maternal problems. If fetal risk is suspected and the clinician wants to rule out meconium, individualize the clinical approach to the patient. If the external electronic monitor is not recording accurately and the information is important in a particular labor, rupture the membranes and apply an internal fetal monitor.

EXAMPLE OF USING MEMBRANE RUPTURE AS A TREATMENT FOR ARRESTED LABOR

A multipara with a normal size fetus was found to be arrested in active phase labor at 5 cm, S−1, vertex LOT, and with membranes intact. How should the membranes be managed?

Comment

One appropriate intervention is to perform AROM. Other possibilities should also be considered. Oxytocin stimulation would be appropriate. Information needed in this case is the quality of the uterine contractions and the amount of patient discomfort.

With all the information, there are several choices. Although AROM is not used in routine fashion, when labor is not progressing it is a treatment choice.

OTHER VARIABLES THAT AFFECT LABOR LENGTH

Vertex position
Clinic pelvimetry
Cervical effacement

Fetal size
The laboring environment

Vertex Position

The effects of posterior and transverse positions of the vertex, of flexion or extension, or even of vertex asynclitism (flexion to right or left) on the length of active phase of labor is not well documented. In fact, the clinician rarely expects a posterior positioned vertex to descend rapidly through the pelvis. The nonanterior diameters are often less efficient delivery mechanisms and require more energy and time for the pelvic muscles to stretch and the vertex to mold, flex, and rotate. When these positions are seen, expect a longer labor course.

Clinical Pelvimetry

Clinical pelvimetry is poorly taught. Some clinicians consider clinical mensuration useless but in this text clinical pelvimetry is presented and suggested for use in an attempt to deliver adequate patient care.

The shape of the maternal pelvis may be such that vertex rotation to an anterior position may not occur until the shape of the pelvis allows rotation to take place. Rotation may take place at a lower pelvic station. In some labors, internal vertex rotation may occur on the perineum. In other patients, the vertex will deliver from a posterior position without rotation. A platypelloid pelvis (characterized in part by a wide sacrosciatic notch) may accommodate a large head more easily in transverse positions.

Clinical pelvimetry should be performed at the first antepartum visit. It may be repeated during labor, but it is not as easily performed at that time. Note also that each time a vaginal examination is performed during labor there may be temporary loss of some vertex station or dilatation.[6] This loss of station may depend on how vigorously the vertex and pelvis are examined.

Cervical Effacement (and Position)

Another clinical variable which is difficult to quantitate is cervical effacement. In one examination an 80% cervical thickness measurement may be reported by examiner as an uneffaced cervix. Some association with labor length and cervical effacement is based on clinical experience; statistics are not available.

In general, the thinner the cervical effacement the more easily and rapidly dilatation will take place. Similarly, the posterior position of the cervix, in contrast to a midpositioned cervix, often foreshadows a longer labor course. Cervical position may be linked with vertex position. The occiput posterior or occiput transverse vertex positions are more common with the posterior cervix. No interventions are suggested. Cervical length or thickness may indicate that labor will be longer or shorter, but it is still a speculation.

Membrane rupture should only be cautiously performed in the presence of a poorly effaced cervix. If the membranes are ruptured, will the presenting part descend and be apposed against the cervix? If following membrane rupture the vertex does not descend against the cervix, difficulty in continuing cervical dilatation may take place. In some cases there may actually be loss of dilatation or regression if membranes are ruptured. It is important to note that this discussion of membrane rupture refers to augmentation or treatment of labor. It does not refer to initiation of labor.

Fetal Size

The larger fetus may be expected to progress through the pelvis more slowly than the average size fetus. There is more vertex for the cervix to dilate and retract over and there is more pelvic and vaginal musculature to be stretched. The smaller fetus with the smaller vertex has a shorter active and second stage of labor. Variable fetal size should be considered in management plans.

Some obstetricians suggest that excessive fetal size is defined as a fetus over 4500 g (9.9 lb) and should lead to an elective cesarean in order to avoid shoulder dystocia.[7] It is true that shoulder dystocia occurs more frequently in large sized infants, however, the majority of large size fetuses deliver normally and without shoulder problems. In fact, the majority of cases of shoulder dystocia occur in normal size fetuses.[7] If labor is continued in the presence of a large fetus, it is appropriate to be less aggressive in management. For example, in a patient with a large fetus and failure to descend to the perineum, the use of midforceps may be associated with shoulder dystocia.

The Patient Care Environment

It is difficult to assess the effect of the patient care environment on the length of active phase labor. The general statements made in Chapter 1 relate to good environmental support, improved patient comfort, removal of anxiety, and the facilitation of relaxation. All of these effects may shorten labor, but how much the environment affects labor is a speculation. The sounds coming from some labor rooms today appear to be symphonies of fetal heart beats.

EXAMPLE OF THE EFFECT OF ENVIRONMENT ON LABOR

A patient in early latent phase labor was observed and monitored for 20 hours. She arrived at 1 cm dilatation and progressed to 6 cm dilated with vertex S–2. She was tolerating labor poorly. There was a protraction of the active phase during the previous 2 hours when she progressed from 5 to 6 cm.

Comment

Any healthy person lying in bed for 20 hours, relatively restricted in movement and always hearing the fetal heart monitor, should be exhausted. This mother needs help. Choices include medication for rest or a regional block. This situation inevitably makes labor tolerance by mother and management by physician more difficult. Perhaps the best cure for this patient would have been to remain home for a longer part of her latent phase.

ACTIVE PHASE INTERVENTIONS

The importance of the labor diagnosis is reemphasized. If progress is continuous and at 1 cm or more each hour, there is usually no need to intervene. If protraction or arrests are present, potential interventions include:

1. Patience
2. Ambulation/position change
3. Medication/analgesia
4. Regional anesthesia
5. Oxytocin
6. Cesarean

In the absence of fetal distress, there is no reason to effect a surgical end to labor without first trying to make a diagnosis. Why is the labor problem happening? Treat the problem. In some cases it is appropriate to end labor prior to an adequate labor trial. On the other hand, many interventions have the potential to increase infant or maternal morbidity. Within the treatments available there is a great amount of latitude.

Risk for infant neurologic injury following abnormal labor dystocia was analyzed at Cleveland Metropolitan General Hospital.[8] Dystocia, defined by protractions and arrests in active labor, and interventions such as oxytocin use, did not correlate with neurologic morbidity in infants 2 years after birth. Neither vaginal nor cesarean birth routes demonstrated improved clinical outcomes or altered neurologic damage.

SUMMARY

1. Active phase labor has three parts.

    a. Accelerative phase

b. Maximum slope of dilatation
c. Decelerative phase

2. In active phase, rate of cervical dilation should equal or exceed 1.2 cm/h for the nullipara and 1.5 cm/h for the multipara.
3. Vertex descent usually takes place late in active phase or during the second stage of labor.
4. Arrests of descent include no change for 1 hour in the nullipara and no change for ½ hour in the multipara.
5. Mean rates of labor do not infer morbidity by themselves; they are guidelines to alert the clinician to intervene.
6. Timely chart notes should document the patient's labor course and the clinician's outcome expectations.
7. Friedman graphs should be plotted in the chart as the patient is being examined during labor.
8. Active phase interventions include:

   a. Patience
   b. Ambulation
   c. Sedation, analgesia
   d. Regional block
   e. AROM
   f. Oxytocin
   g. Cesarean

9. Forceps use should be reserved for second stage interventions.

REFERENCES

1. Shiono PH, McNellis D, Rhoads GG: Reasons for the rising cesarean delivery rates. Obstet Gynecol 1987;69:696–700.
2. Peisner DB, Rosen MG: The latent phase of labor in normal patients: a reassessment. Obstet Gynecol 1985;66:644–648.
3. O'Driscoll K, Meagher D: Active Management of Labour. London, Philadelphia, Toronto, WB Saunders, 1980, p 106.
4. Cohen WA, Friedman ER: Management of Labor. Baltimore, University Park Press, 1983, Chapter 2.
5. Sokol RJ, Nussbaum RS, Chik L, Rosen MG: Computer diagnosis of labor progression. V. Reliability of a subroutine for evaluating station and descent of the fetal presenting part during labor. J Reprod Med 1974;13:183–186.
6. Acker DB, Sachs BP, Friedman EA: Risk factors for shoulder dystocia. Obstet Gynecol 1985;66:762–768.
7. Bottoms SF, Sokol RJ, Rosen MG: Short arrest of dilatation: a risk for maternal and fetal infant morbidity. Am J Obstet Gynecol 1981;140:108–116.
8. Rosen MG: Dystocia, arrest disorders and infant brain damage. Obstet Gynecol 1989;74 (in press).
9. Sokol RJ, Stoikof J, Chik L, Rosen MG: Normal and abnormal labor progress. I. A quantitative assessment and survey of the literature. J Reprod Med 1977;18:47–53.

Chapter 8

Second Stage of Labor

OVERVIEW

In Chapter 7, active phase labor was characterized in terms of medical management. As a surgical procedure, the cesarean was considered only after medical management had been tried and failed. In marked contrast, historically, the second stage of labor has involved a large surgical component. Although most fetuses deliver spontaneously, second stage labor interventions include the use of forceps, the vacuum extractor, and the cesarean. It is in the second stage of labor that physical trauma to mother and fetus may take place. The second stage of labor is a time when both the patient and the clinician may be physically and emotionally exhausted, and when interventions to end labor are expected.

The second stage of labor begins with full cervical dilatation and ends with fetal birth. The interventions for second stage labor have important historical precedents which presage today's reasons for clinical care.

OBJECTIVES

At the conclusion of this chapter, the clinician should be able to:

1. Define the second stage of labor
2. Understand the historical precedents for various interventions
3. Understand the clinical problems leading to prolonged second stage labor
4. Determine appropriate medical and surgical interventions for the second stage of labor
5. Define the pathologies consequent to second stage labor interventions

EVOLUTION OF SECOND STAGE LABOR MANAGEMENT

In one of the more famous obstetrical stories, Sir Eardley Holland, as quoted by Hellman and Prystowsky,[1] described the death of Princess Charlotte following what was obviously an arrest in labor. Sir Richard Croft, the princess's physician, was faced with the dilemma of intervening to save the life of Princess Charlotte and destroying the fetus (the future king of England), or performing a cesarean to save the fetus, most probably leading to the death of the princess (the future queen of England). Neither treatment forecast a satisfactory outcome, and, in the dilemma created by the two choices, Sir Richard chose to do nothing. Ultimately, both members of the royal family, prince and future king, died. Sir Richard committed suicide sometime later, perhaps in remorse over this tragic outcome. outcome.

The introduction of the use of forceps gave obstetricians an alternative to the cesarean which, at that time, inevitably led to the mother's death. Appropriate forceps use became an obstetrical debate more than 100 years ago and still continues today. Soon after their introduction, forceps use became the hallmark of the obstetrician—which separated him from the midwife. In contrast, today midforceps use in second stage labor carries with it an almost unspoken stigma and is rapidly becoming lost as an obstetrical skill. Neither extreme appears appropriate.

In 1820 Merriman[1] (again quoted by Hellman and Prystowsky[1]) wrote, "Forceps shall never be applied until the ear of the child has been within reach of the operator's fingers for at least 6 hours." Thus the 6-hour rule was introduced. Other rules were soon to follow. Even today clinicians often quote and act according to a 2-hour rule, the origin of which Hellman and Prystowsky also describe.[1] Most clinicians practicing today accept the fact that the second stage should be no longer than 2 hours or it is abnormal and should be ended. Shortening of the second stage of labor to the 2-hour rule was brought about by Delee.[1] He urged the application of "prophylactic forceps" in a paper read before the American Gynecological Society in 1920.[1]

The medical value of the 2-hour rule was studied for morbidity by Hellman and Prystowsky[1] at the Johns Hopkins Hospital between 1937 and 1949. During that interval prophylactic forceps were used to shorten the second stage of labor. About 3% of all labors exceeded a 3-hour second stage with a median second stage duration for multiparas of 20 minutes, and 50 minutes for primiparas. The authors observed that prolongation of the second stage was associated with increased postpartum hemorrhage, puerperal infection, and infant morbidity. This classic paper also foreshadowed Friedman's later studies about labor and delivery. The authors noted an association between first stage labor abnormalities and second stage problems, and also observed the effect of posterior vertex positions on labor length.[1]

Evaluation of the link between labor abnormalities and fetal and neonatal morbidity continued in more current studies by Bottoms et al,[2] although this retrospective review did not distinguish whether fetal complications were already present and produced neonatal morbidity, or whether the labor abnormalities produced the wastage. It was clear that significant differences in neonatal neurologic morbidity were not found when both occurred either by cesarean or vaginal route following protractions or arrest. Wayne Cohen[3] studying the lengths of second stage labors, found no increase in depressed Apgar scores or neonatal morbidity in second stages prolonged beyond 3 hours. He did notice that there was continuing evidence for increased maternal postpartum hemorrhage and infection, as Hellman and Prystowsky had noted many years earlier. It is notable that the Bottoms report was followed by a long-term study by Rosen et al that confirmed the neonatal study.[4] This report came from an obstetrical service where midforceps use was rare, and may reflect the separation of a prolonged second stage of labor from a difficult forceps birth. The confounding variables of prolonged second stage labor, or fetal distress, cannot easily be separated from the effects of midforceps applications when attempting to determine later neurologic risk for the infant. This area of dystocia and forceps is reviewed again in Chapter 10. Thus, although we define second stage labor as onset with full dilatation and there are mean values to describe average lengths, an arbitrary rule by number, such as the 2-hour rule, is not acceptable as a concept to end labor.

DEFINITION OF SECOND STAGE LABOR (Table 8.1)

Classic descriptors may be used for the definition of the second stage of labor. Second stage labor begins at full cervical dilatation and ends with the

TABLE 8.1 Second Stage Labor Definitions

Failed	No descent is noted from time patient is first examined
Protraction (in the 2nd stage)	Nullipara: Descent <1 cm/h
	Multipara: Descent <2 cm/h
Arrest (in the 2nd stage)	No change *after* descent has begun
	Nullipara: 1 h
	Multipara: 30 min

Modified from Friedman.

birth of the neonate. If there is pathology in the second stage of labor, the vertex either does not descend (failed descent), descent progresses too slowly (protraction of descent), or descent stops after starting (arrest of descent).

The use of time limits and rules are guidelines for interventions. Morbidity cannot be predicted either in long or short second stage labor. If, as one would logically believe, there is some point beyond which the second stage of labor becomes morbid, that length of time is not known to the clinician. The 2-hour rule appears arbitrary and often too short. A 3- or 4-hour rule cannot be made without data. In fact, many clinicians do follow patients in second stage labor for 3 and 4 hours in the presence of normal fetal monitoring of term infants and when descent is slow but continuing.

CHARACTER OF NORMAL DESCENT DURING SECOND STAGE LABOR

Descent is progressive and usually begins later in the active phase. More multiparas are unengaged at labor onset and may stay that way until the second stage is well underway. Dystocia associated with a mismatch of fetus with pelvis size cannot be accurately assessed until the patient is well into the active or second stage of labor.

The nullipara usually enters labor at a lower pelvic station. Descent may not begin until the second stage is established. While it is taught that most nulliparas will demonstrate vertex engagement at labor onset, that dictum more correctly refers to the patient's perceived signs of "lightening" and the abdominal examination conducted with Leopold's maneuvers, which may confirm that the vertex is relatively well placed within the pelvis. On vaginal examination it is often found that the presenting part is still above the ischial spines. Further vaginal descent will begin to take place after labor onset and often not until the decelerative portion of the active phase or the second stage of labor.

The second stage of labor tests pelvic capacity for fetal size. In most patients, irrespective of pelvic size, the cervix will continue to dilate around the fetal head even though descent does not take place. The diagnosis of cephalopelvic disproportion cannot be made with accuracy until full or almost full cervical dilatation has been reached. Perhaps in a very small number of patients clinical pelvimetry can predict absolute disproportion; however, few patients have that small or distorted a pelvis so that the clinician may say the fetus will not deliver vaginally.

FACTORS ASSOCIATED WITH ABNORMALITIES OF SECOND STAGE LABORS

Active Phase Abnormality

Active phase labor abnormalities show consistent associations with problems in the second stage of labor. This is in contrast to latent phase abnormalities which do not predict labor problems.[5] Protractions and arrests in the active phase may be associated with descent problems.[6] If active phase labor abnormalities have already been noted, anticipate second stage abnormalities.

Maternal and Fetal Size and Clinical Pelvimetry

Maternal size, particularly for the very short patient (under 5 ft tall), is a consideration. But even in the short mother, clinical estimates are rarely indications to prevent a trial of labor. Maternal size along with clinical pelvimetry estimates alert the clinician to a potential for labor problems, which allows for earlier intervention than in a labor where there appear to be no factors suggesting pelvic disproportion.

Excessive maternal weight (with respect to height) should also be listed as a risk factor.

Fetal size over 4,000 or 4,500 g may be useful in raising suspicion that second stage labor may be prolonged. Size may be a concern; yet, the majority of large fetuses deliver normally. Thus the clinical impression is only additional information to be processed and used in the management plan. Excessive maternal weight gain is associated with increased fetal size.

Increased fetal size is associated with increased maternal prepregnancy weight and also with excessive weight gain during pregnancy. Therefore, in the presence of these maternal risk factors, carefully document fetal size.

The clinical maternal and fetal size risk factors provide guides which caution the clinician to avoid aggressive interventions. Some of these conditions include: a large fetus, an obese mother, a postdates mother with a known large fetus, a diabetic mother, or a preexisting active phase abnormality. The clinician may consider medical interventions (time, analgesia, oxytocin) but good judgment dictates earlier termination in the management of these labors. It would be of value to supplement the clinician's examination with ultrasonographic evidence of fetal size near term. Be wary of forceps use in these situations.

CLINICAL INTERVENTIONS IN SECOND STAGE LABOR

Possible interventions of second stage labor include:

1. Patience
2. Ambulation

3. Stimulation (oxytocin)
4. Analgesia
5. Regional anesthesia
6. Cesarean
7. Forceps/vacuum

The decrease in the use of all forceps during the last 25 years has been appropriate. Labor should be completed without excessive force. A difficult labor, terminated by use of difficult forceps, is associated with increased risk for fetal and maternal trauma.

EXAMPLE OF MORE TIME GIVEN FOR THE SECOND STAGE (Figure 8.1)

A normal nullipara at term with an estimated 7-lb fetus has been in labor for 12 hours and has been fully dilated for 1 hour. The vertex is LOT. During the last 3 hours the vertex has progressed from station −1 to station 0.

Comment

This is not an uncommon clinical finding during the second stage. By definition, this is a protraction of descent. However, in the OT position anticipate slower descent as vertex flexion, molding, and then vertex rotation must take place. Watchful waiting is appropriate as long as progress continues. An arbitrary 2-hour rule is not acceptable. An alternative plan for this patient could include ambulation. During ambulation monitor the fetal heart each 5 minutes with auscultation or a Doptone device. The use of oxytocin is acceptable if it is felt that the contractions are not as strong as they should be. The use of analgesia or anesthesia is appropriate if maternal pain or poor relaxation is a consideration. Forceps intervention or a cesarean are not considered at this time. The vertex may not be engaged despite the molded vertex which is felt at the ischial spines.

Anesthesia or Analgesia

Pain relief with the use of regional anesthesia, such as the epidural or regional block, will provide relaxation of pelvic muscles. Some clinicians would argue that epidural anesthesia increases the use of forceps; that descent and vertex rotations may not take place as easily. That question cannot be resolved. Do not routinely use regional anesthesia. When there is the need for pain relief or failure to rotate or descend is present, regional anesthesia is another therapeutic choice. If failure to rotate or descend follows an earlier regional block, it can be overcome with oxytocin stimulation, or by allowing the anesthetic to "wear off."

It is impossible to predict the effect of pain relief therapy. The clinician has this option for treatment which is reversible and incurs little risk.

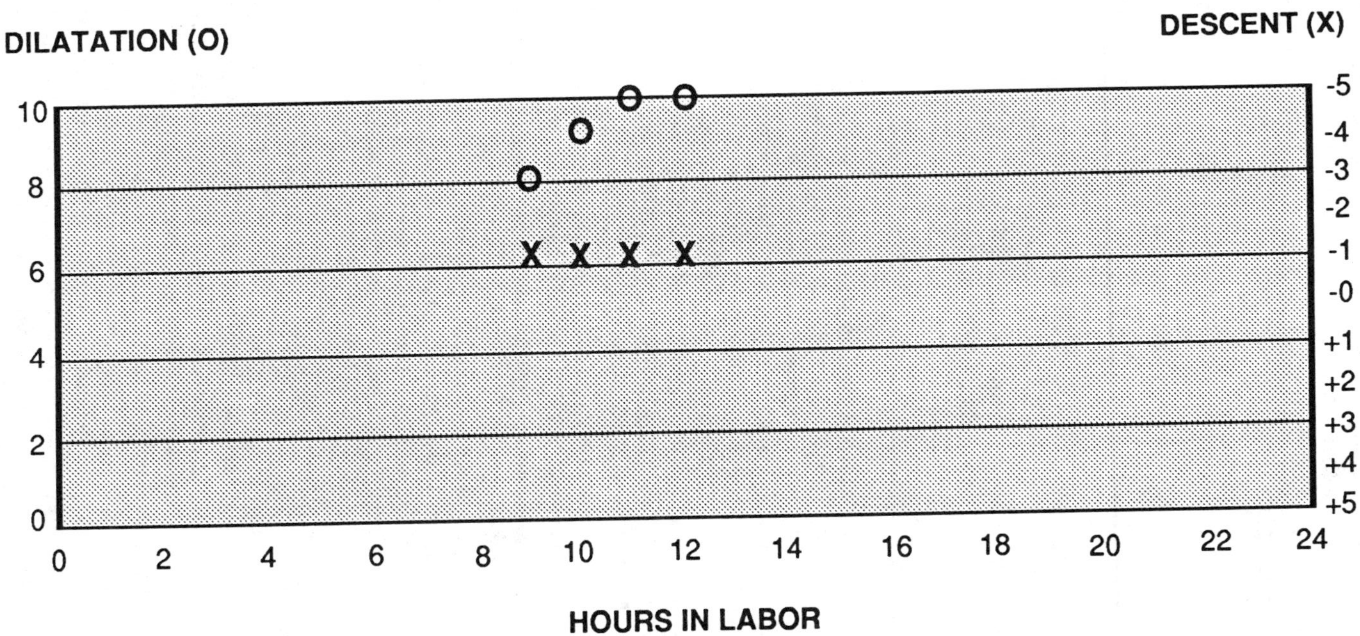
DILATATION (O)
DESCENT (X)
10
8
6
4
2
0
-5
-4
-3
-2
-1
-0
+1
+2
+3
+4
+5
0
2
4
6
8
10
12
14
16
18
20
22
24
HOURS IN LABOR

FIGURE 8.1

Rapid cervical dilatation and vertex descent may follow medication use. Rapid dilatation and descent have also slowed following this same intervention. Thus, the medication use should not be routine, it should be used selectively and for pain.

Oxytocin

On the fetal monitoring tracing, bell-shaped contractions may be apparent. Yet the expected cervical dilatation and vertex descent may not take place. Even if palpation indicates adequate contractions at the bedside, cervical dilatation and descent may not take place. The final guide for patient care is the rate of cervical dilation in active phase labor and vertex descent in second stage labor. If, after starting oxytocin, descent does not take place in a progressive manner, disproportion must be considered and new interventions are indicated.

EXAMPLE OF OXYTOCIN SUPPLEMENT FOR FAILURE TO DESCEND DURING THE SECOND STAGE (Figure 8.2)

In a multipara, following 8 hours of progressive labor, epidural anesthesia was administered at full cervical dilatation and the vertex at station −2 in the LOT position. During the next 2 hours the vertex failed to descend. The fetal heart rate tracing continued to display normal findings. Because the fear of recurrence of the labor pain was an important consideration for this patient, rather than discontinue the analgesia the obstetrician used oxytocin stimulation.

Comment

Oxytocin use was appropriate in this case and is appropriate in the presence of protractions or arrests of descent. Continuing observation must take place when these "next steps" are considered. In this case, although contractions appeared adequate, no progress was being made. Judgment involves watching the fetal heart rate to be certain that the addition of oxytocin does not lead to deprivation of supply to the fetus as may be demonstrated by periodic delayed decelerations or diminished heart rate beat-to-beat variability. Frequency of contractions and adequate return to normal pressure baselines between contractions is reassuring. However, prolonged use of oxytocin without progress is to be discouraged.

The clinician should always consider using oxytocin in the presence of what would appear to be good uterine contractions. Contraction shape or perceived intensity is not satisfactory unless progress is made. In this situation, following the use of oxytocin expect progressive descent in 1 hour. If no progress occurs, the failure to descend may not be due to the forces of labor; look for other causes, such as fetal size, vertex position, or pelvic capacity. If slow progress continues and no monitoring abnormalities are present, oxytocin use may continue. Be cautious before considering any forceps as an intervention in difficult second stages of labor. Try to avoid midforceps as an intervention. At a point when descent has been a second stage labor problem move to cesarean rather than midforceps, even if the

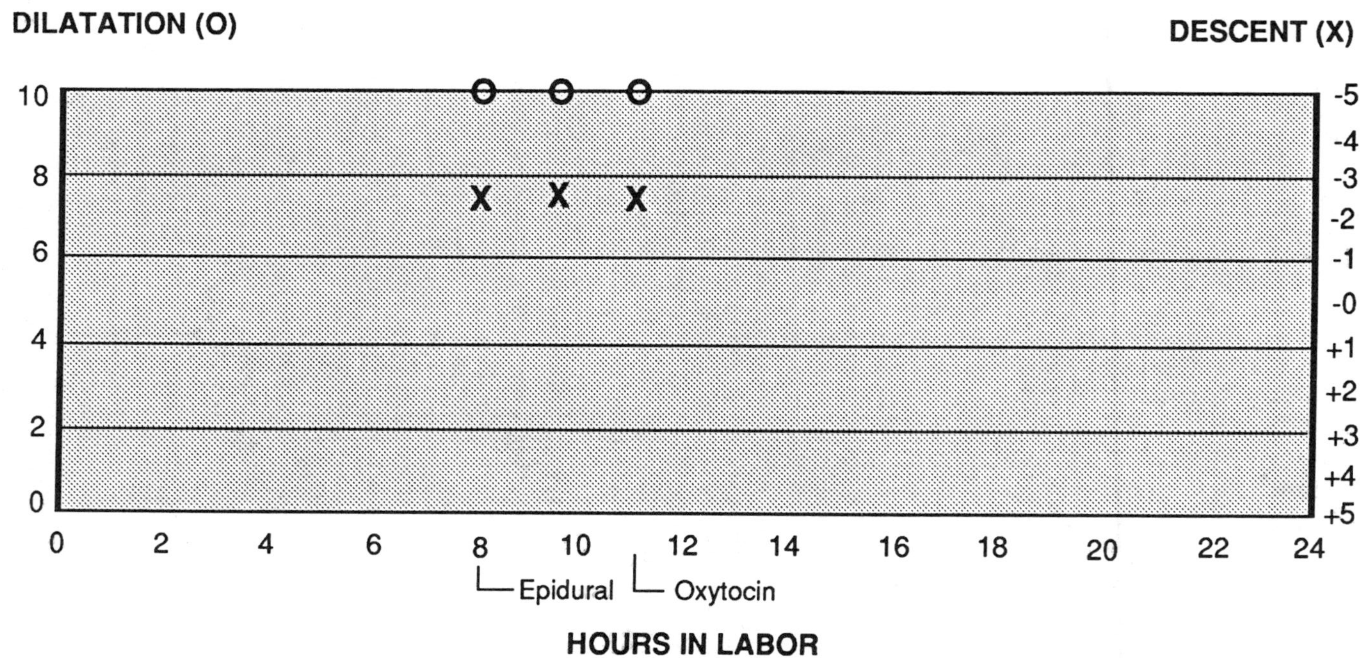
DILATATION (O)
DESCENT (X)
10
8
6
4
2
0
-5
-4
-3
-2
-1
-0
+1
+2
+3
+4
+5
0
2
4
6
8
10
12
14
16
18
20
22
24
Epidural
Oxytocin
HOURS IN LABOR

FIGURE 8.2

head has become engaged. After 3 or more hours in second stage labor, the vertex, with its molding and caput, is probably not as low in the pelvis as it may appear. Avoid what may be anticipated as difficult midforceps.

EXAMPLE OF A LONG SECOND STAGE AND OXYTOCIN USE FOLLOWED BY PROGRESS (Figure 8.3)

After 10 hours of labor, a P2 G3 mother was fully dilated and at station +1 for 2 hours. The vertex was OA. An arrest of descent was diagnosed at station +1. The monitoring tracing displayed uterine contractions every 3 to 4 minutes with occasional coupling of contractions. Oxytocin stimulation was instituted. The vertex descended during the next hour to station +2.

Comment

Although the second stage was 3 hours in length, progress was taking place. In the absence of electronic fetal monitoring abnormalities, continued stimulation was reasonable. Midforceps use for slow progress at this time would be inappropriate. Avoid getting involved in the sequence of an arrest followed by oxytocin use with some progress, and then followed by midforceps application. As noted earlier, there is no guide to determine how long to continue the labor before giving up on the vaginal birth. The decision as to when a cesarean should be performed must be individualized. If progress continues, the decision may be made to allow more time in labor. If progress stops while using oxytocin, or if progress does not take place, cesarean birth is the choice. There are no hourly rules. The 2-hour rule is too arbitrary. Judgment is needed. In contrast to the term infant, in the presence of fetal distress or a low-birth-weight fetus, interventions would be more rapid.

EXAMPLE OF AN ARREST OF DESCENT AND THE 2-HOUR RULE (Figure 8.4)

After a 14-hour labor, a P0 G1 mother with vertex OP was at station +2 and fully dilated. No change in station had taken place for 2 hours. She was stimulated with oxytocin. During the next 2 hours vaginal examinations confirmed increasing caput and molding. Although it appeared that descent was occurring on vaginal examination, the obstetrician, allowing for the change in size and shape of the vertex, felt descent was minimal or absent and chose to perform a cesarean rather than persist.

Comment

In the absence of fetal emergencies, do not use forceps between station 0 and +2 in a five-station pelvis. Try other measures such as time, regional anesthesia, or use of oxytocin, although failure to observe progress with oxytocin use leaves few options. The length of time observation may be continued is uncertain. Most clinicians stop oxytocin use in active or second stage labor in the absence of observed progress after 1 or at most 2 hours of a trial. This clinical situation, with vertex engaged, takes place relatively infrequently. Usually, the vertex arrests at higher stations.

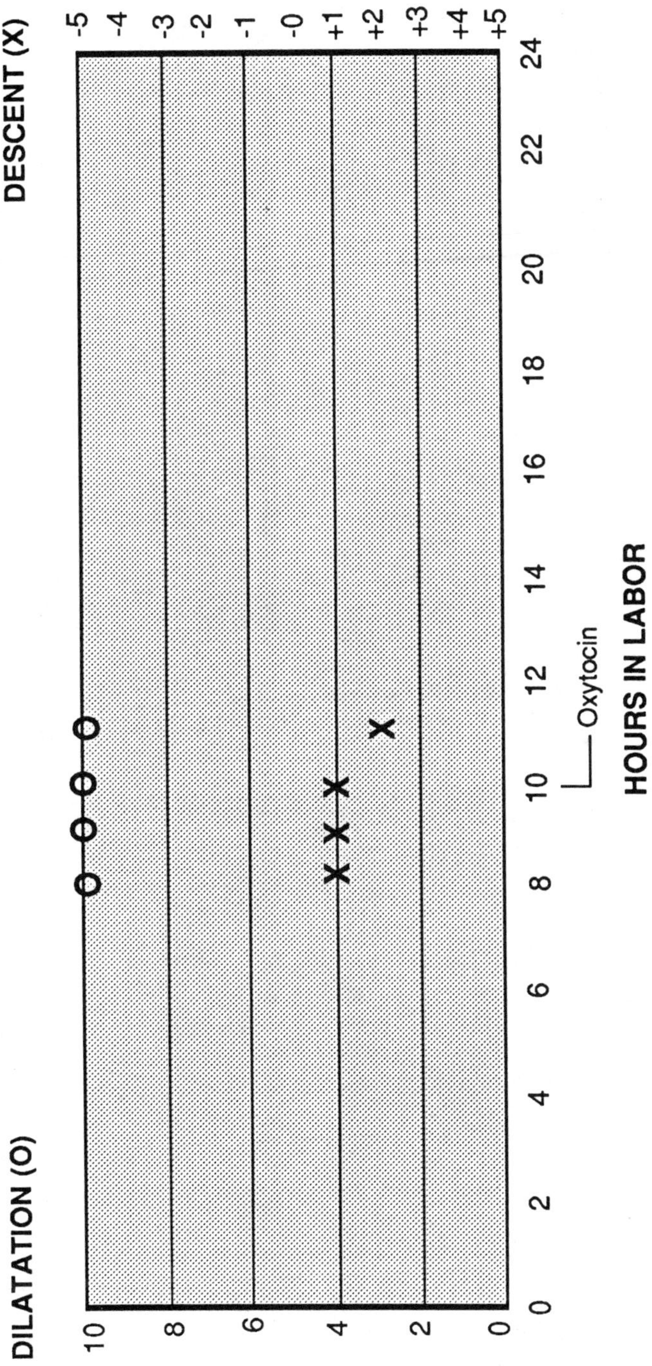
DILATATION (O)
DESCENT (X)
10
8
6
4
2
0
-5
-4
-3
-2
-1
-0
+1
+2
+3
+4
+5
0
2
4
6
8
10
12
14
16
18
20
22
24
Oxytocin
HOURS IN LABOR

FIGURE 8.3

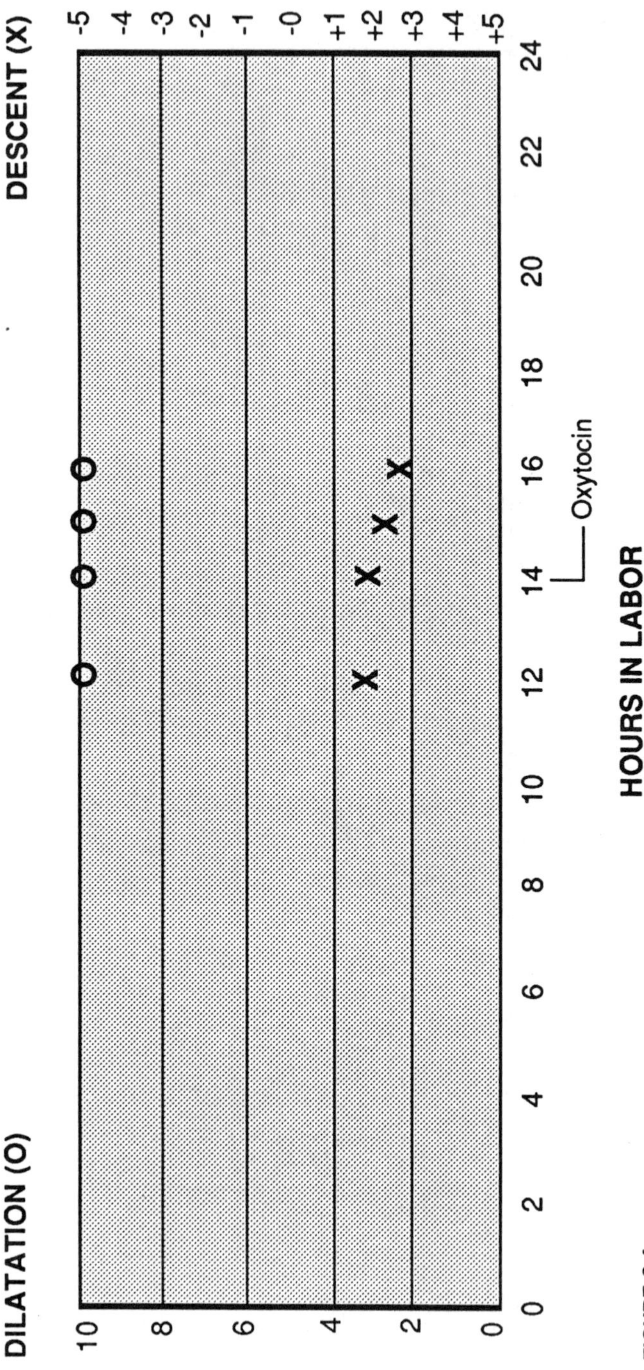
DILATATION (O)
DESCENT (X)
10
8
6
4
2
0
-5
-4
-3
-2
-1
-0
+1
+2
+3
+4
+5
0
2
4
6
8
10
12
14
16
18
20
22
24
Oxytocin
HOURS IN LABOR

FIGURE 8.4

When the fetus is in the pelvis at this level, expect continuing descent to take place. However, in posterior positions much more vertex molding takes place and that takes time. Despite the patient being haltered with a monitor and oxytocin in the venous lines, maternal position may be changed, and the patient may even be ambulated. If ambulation is used, monitoring (telemetry, if available, or Doptone) must continue. If oxytocin is being used, monitoring should be continuous. Another intervention to be considered in low-station-descent arrests is epidural anesthesia along with oxytocin augmentation. Pelvic relaxation may facilitate vertex descent.

Forceps/Vacuum Extraction

Forceps and vacuum extraction are additional therapeutic interventions for use in the second stage of labor. Forceps use should be defined and classified by station. A complete discussion of forceps use is covered in Chapters 11 and 12.

EXAMPLE OF FORCEPS USE TO SHORTEN SECOND STAGE LABOR

A nulliparous mother was exhausted following a 20-hour labor. The vertex was at station +5 in OA position. The vertex was seen on the perineum without spreading the labia with each contraction. The mother could not push out the fetus. A low forceps was effected for maternal indications.

Comment

The use of forceps from low station to shorten the second stage is acceptable if the mother's situation calls for their use. Some clinicians would describe this as an outlet forceps and confine the definition for low forceps to station +4. As noted in Chapter 12 classifying forceps by station and rotation adds more information and removes the categories low, mid, and outlet forceps which have varying definitions to obstetricians.

EXAMPLE OF MATERNAL EXHAUSTION IN A VERTEX OCCIPUT POSTERIOR (VOP) POSITION

A nulliparous mother had been actively "pushing" during the second stage of labor for the past 2 hours. Inspection of the perineum revealed dilatation of the vagina with each contraction, but the vertex could not actually be seen by the examiner without further labial separation. The vaginal examination revealed molding and caput with the vertex at station +4, and in an LOP position.

Comment

The reason the vagina separated and yet the vertex was not visualized without spreading the labia was that in the OP or OT positions, wider diameters of the vertex separate the vaginal walls before crowning is seen. Allowing more time would be effective. If the patient is taken to the delivery room at this point without crowning taking place, the forceps birth will be more difficult than expected. Although, because of the molding, the vertex feels lower in station, this vertex is more likely at station +2 or +3. The vertex is deliverable, but it will require more traction force. By definition, this is a midforceps delivery if the station is +4 or higher. Along with other medical interventions, use of regional anesthesia such as epidural blockage may facilitate vertex descent while preserving the ability to "push."

STATION +2/+3

A vertex at station +2 to +3 (of five pelvic stations) should be expected to deliver vaginally. This may not always occur spontaneously. If a second stage descent abnormality follows regional block during a normal labor, several therapeutic choices are available (time, oxytocin, or allowing medication to wear off). In the absence of fetal distress, forceps use and the cesarean should be deferred. In fact, it may be difficult to deliver a station +3 vertex by cesarean because of the depth of the vertex in the pelvis.

Stations +2 and +3 contrast with lower pelvic stations (remember, in this text five stations to the pelvis are used); therapeutic interventions are always more worrisome at this point of labor. Following a protraction of the active phase or in association with an arrest of descent, the decision to use forceps should be most cautious. With skills that should be acquired during resident education, vaginal birth in most cases can be effected with forceps. However, once a protraction or arrest of descent has taken place, be wary of forceps use. They will usually be more difficult and may presage a larger fetus or difficulty with the shoulders.

EXAMPLE OF ACTIVE AND SECOND STAGE LABOR ABNORMALITIES (Figure 8.5)

A multiparous patient had a latent phase of 12 hours. During active phase labor she arrested for 3 hours, at station −2 and 7 cm cervical dilatation. The fetus was normal in size and the contractions appeared adequate. The patient was exhausted. She was given 50 mg of meperidine intravenously. At the same time augmentation of labor with oxytocin resulted in slow progress. Three hours after oxytocin use, the patient was fully dilated and at station +2. Thus this situation is a long active phase with slow progress. Two hours later dilatation was at station +3.

Comment

In this case, beware of the use of midforceps. The cesarean is a prudent decision. This has been a difficult labor with active and second stage pathology. Despite what

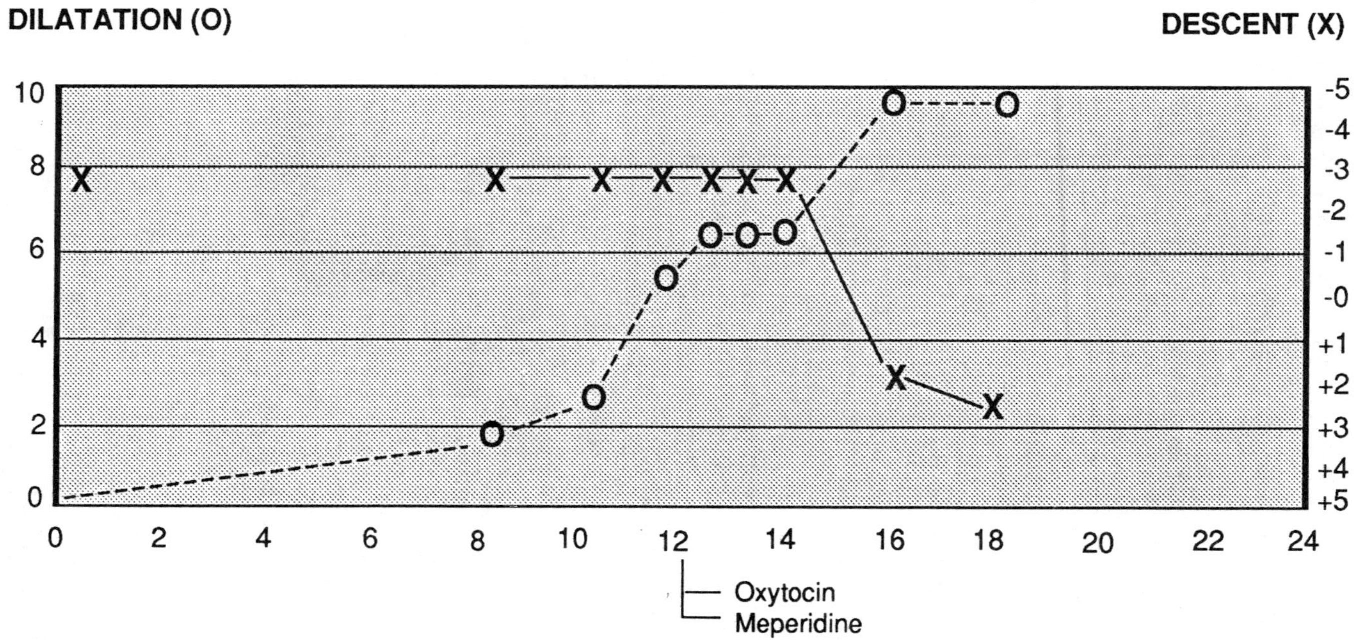
DILATATION (O)
DESCENT (X)
10
8
6
4
2
0
-5
-4
-3
-2
-1
-0
+1
+2
+3
+4
+5
0
2
4
6
8
10
12
14
16
18
20
22
24
Oxytocin
Meperidine
HOURS IN LABOR

FIGURE 8.5

the clinician may think he or she feels allowing for caput and molding, the vertex is probably not at station +3. In most examples such as this, once oxytocin has begun, consider also the use of regional anesthesia to provide muscle relaxation and pain relief.

It is important to have neurologic data relating to midforceps use as assessed by each station of the pelvis. Friedman's data derived from the Collaborative Cerebral Palsy Study in the 1960s and Dierker and Rosen's data from Cleveland Metropolitan General Hospital in the 1970s suggest different conclusions about forceps use and will be discussed in Chapter 11 on midforceps. Midforceps use in the presence of protractions or arrests are not easily advocated. Even if the operator believes he or she is skillful enough to effect vaginal delivery, caution is advised as a protraction or arrest in the second stage may foreshadow more difficulty in the delivery.

USE OF FETAL MONITORING WITH ACTIVE AND SECOND STAGE ABNORMALITIES

The patient without antepartum risk whose labor progresses normally need not be electronically monitored if the fetal heart rate can be auscultated each 30 minutes during the latent phase and each 15 minutes during the active phase. If labor progression during active and second stage does not occur at the expected rate and intervention is considered, electronic monitoring should be instituted. When oxytocin is used, both external and internal monitoring modes are acceptable. These cautionary measures regarding monitoring are taken with the understanding of both the benefits and the limitations of monitoring.

For example, it is accepted that too frequent contractions from oxytocin use may be associated with delayed decelerations or fetal bradycardia. The visually displayed patterns allow for quicker diagnosis and treatment. However, the absence of fetal heart rate abnormalities, for example, in the presence of an arrest of labor in the active phase, or an arrest of descent during the second stage of labor, does not always portray intracerebral events secondary to the difficult labor which may foreshadow cerebral injury. Thus, the clinician must rely on prudent judgment in treating the problems. Stated differently we do not have information which allows for rules to be set on the length of time one should allow for labor or the use of oxytocin. One cannot depend on electronic fetal monitoring for these answers.

Throughout this book references have been made to the too frequent use of the cesarean during the latent and active phases of labor. An adequate trial of labor in order to test pelvic capacity has been the major theme. However, cesareans performed during the second stage of labor are not usually criticized. Time for allowing the vertex to mold, flex, rotate, and descend is continuously stressed. Second stage is not the heart of the cesarean debate. The clinician may choose to perform a cesarean in the presence of an arrest of descent at station +3 based on training and recent clinical experience. Another clinician may choose forceps based on different training. The high cesarean birthrate is less associated with the use of the cesarean during the second stage of labor. If an adequate trial of labor has been given, the cesarean avoids Sir Richard's dilemma of not intervening.

Strict adherence to the 2-hour rule is not valid and must be replaced by clinical judgment. The absence of observed fetal distress suggests that neuropathology does not follow unless a traumatic delivery takes place, but the monitor is limited in this area. Stated conversely, more time allowed for delivery without forceps does not appear to be traumatic.

SUMMARY

1. The second stage of labor begins with full dilatation and ends with birth.
2. Descent of the vertex usually begins late during the active phase of labor and continues through the second stage of labor.
3. Pathologies of second stage labor include:

   Arrest of descent (no progress): > 1 h nullipara
> 30 min multipara

   Protraction of descent: < 1 cm/h nullipara
< 2 cm/h multipara

   Failed descent: No descent during labor
4. Treatment interventions for second stage include:
   a. Patience
   b. Ambulation
   c. Analgesia and anesthesia
   d. Stimulation
   e. Low forceps, midforceps, vacuum extraction
   f. Cesarean
5. Second stage pathologies are associated with delay or failure of the vertex to rotate, descend, or flex well. Fetuses in these positions often do not conform to the expected labor patterns.
6. Compared with other stages of labor, it is in the second stage of labor that pelvic capacity is tested.

7. Clinical judgment involved in choosing when and how to terminate second stage labors is difficult to define and may be considered the "art" of patient care. The relationship between neurologic morbidity, abnormal labor, and birth route choice is still being debated.
8. Arbitrary termination of second stage labor at the end of 2 hours is inappropriate when slow progress in descent continues.
9. Following abnormal second stage labors, midforceps should be used infrequently and with caution.

REFERENCES

1. Hellman L, Prystowsky H: The duration of the second stage of labor. Am J Obstet Gynecol 1952;63:1223–1233.
2. Bottoms SF, Hirsh JJ, Sokol RJ: Medical management of arrest disorders of labor: A current overview. Am J Obstet Gynecol 1989;156:935–939.
3. Cohen W: The influence of the duration of the second stage labor on perinatal outcome and puerperal morbidity. Obstet Gynecol 1977;49:266–269.
4. Rosen MG, Debanne SM, Thompson K: Arrest disorders and infant brain damage. Obstet Gynecol 1989;74:321–324.
5. Peisner DB, Rosen MG: The latent phase of labor: a reassessment. Obstet Gynecol 1985;66:644–648.
6. Friedman EM, Sachtleben MR: Station of the presentation: Part V. Protracted descent patterns. Obstet Gynecol 1970;36:558–567.

Chapter 9

Management of Active Phase and Second Stage Labor Abnormalities

OVERVIEW

The active phase of labor is the portion of labor in which most obstetrical clinical management skills are called upon. In one management position the cesarean may be appropriate and will terminate the labor without continuing the physician's anxieties, which are generated in caring for a patient when labor is not proceeding well. In contrast, management of a nonsurgical nature takes more time, occurs in an environment of increasing patient and physician discomfort, and raises fetal risk questions which are ill-defined. For example, it is not known how long active phase labor may persist or how much molding or pressure on the fetal vertex can be sustained during second stage labor without increasing the risk for fetal morbidity.

The neglected and prolonged labors of the past were traumatic to mother and fetus. As a guide, a prolonged labor may be defined as a labor which extends more than two standard deviations from an arithmetic mean of all labors. The numbers are not synonymous with brain damage. No study has shown that a 3-hour second stage labor is more morbid than a 2-hour second stage labor.

In this chapter two previously described concepts are reintroduced: orderly *diagnostic evaluation* of the clinical problem, and *therapeutic intervention* for treatment of the laboring patient. The goal is to be sure that all interventions are considered before failure of vaginal birth may occur.

OBJECTIVES

At the conclusion of this chapter, the clinician should be able to:

1. Demonstrate an orderly process for evaluating the diagnostic problems of the patient in active and second stage labor
2. Describe the complete set of therapeutic interventions available for treatment of active labor patients
3. Document reasons for decision choices for the individual patient
4. Complete a proper chart note describing the process.

DEFINITIONS OF ACTIVE PHASE LABOR

Warning: The rates and mean values are guidelines to clinical interventions. If repetition is one characteristic of teaching, then this warning cannot be repeated too often. The numbers used to define normal labor by themselves are not indicative of brain damage. They are guides to alert the clinician that a diagnosis and some new treatment may be needed.

Active phase labor is defined as a rate of cervical dilatation which equals or exceeds:

1.2 cm/h in the nullipara

1.5 cm/h in the multipara

The transition from latent to active phase may be confusing. Is the patient still in latent phase or is the rate of cervical dilatation rapid enough to be called active phase?

If the clinician is uncertain, 5 cm of dilatation is considered to be active labor. Many patients reach active phase dilatation rates at 3 or 4 cm of cervical dilatation and may enter active phase labor earlier.[1,2]

TRANSITION PHASE

The transition time from latent to active phase is depicted in Figure 9.1 at A. It is inconstant in time and simply a change in the rate of dilatation from slow to more rapid.

1. When in doubt treat as if in active labor.
2. When at 5 cm treat as active labor.
3. Note the shaded block in Figure 9.1 at A may occur earlier than 3 cm or later than 5 cms of dilatation.

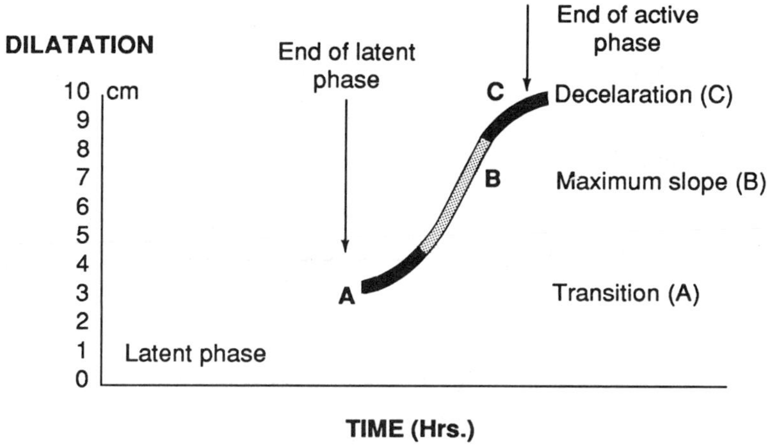

FIGURE 9.1

MAXIMUM RATE OF DILATATION (Figure 9.1 at B)

The area described as maximum rate of dilatation is seen in Figure 9.1 at B (dotted line). At this point in labor, since there is good indication as to how fast a cervix will dilate by comparing the dilatation examinations of the patient, the clinician may anticipate the length of the labor.

EXAMPLE OF EARLY ACTIVE PHASE LABOR ONSET

A patient entered the hospital with cervix at 1 cm dilatation and 50% effacement. Between the next two pelvic examinations within 1 hour, the cervix changed from 1 cm to 3 cm of dilatation and was now 80% effaced.

Comment

By definition, whether nullipara or multipara, a dilatation rate of 2 cm/h means that the patient is in the active phase of labor. If the rate of dilation were to slow or stop during the next several hours, the labor diagnosis would be an arrest in active phase. The diagnosis would not be latent phase labor.

EXAMPLE OF USING CERVICAL DILATATION RATE TO PREDICT THE COURSE OF LABOR

A multipara was examined at 4 AM and found to be 3 cm dilated. At 5 AM she was 5 cm dilated.

Comment

Obviously the patient is in active labor. Using a cervical dilation rate of 1.5 cm/h, expect this patient to be fully dilated between 9 AM and 10 AM (or earlier). Adding 1 hour (expected) for the second stage in a multipara provides a good estimate of when delivery may occur. It is useful to evaluate labor and predict when delivery is likely to take place. If the vertex is in transverse or posterior position, the prediction may be altered and slower progress expected. Other variables, such as fetal size and pelvic station, allow individualized patient considerations.

DECELERATIVE PHASE (Figure 9.1 at C)

Despite the previous example, the rate of cervical dilation may slow towards the end of active phase dilation. This is normal and described as the decelerative phase.

Towards the end of the active phase two changes may be seen which alter patient progress. They are in the decelerative phase of labor and the descent of vertex. Some obstetricians would argue that there is no decelerative phase or slowdown in normal labor progression. Others would disagree (see Chapter 7). In posterior or transverse positions of the vertex, rotation of the vertex may not take place as rapidly as expected. Full cervical dilation may not be present until after the rotation. This may take more time; thus, deceleration or slowing of progress is seen at higher pelvic stations. The vertex more often has not rotated to an anterior position. In contrast, in anterior positions of the vertex, dilation may proceed more rapidly.

EXAMPLE OF PERSISTENT 9-cm CERVIX IN POSTERIOR POSITION

A multiparous patient was noted on vaginal examination to be in vertex OP station 0, at 7 AM, and unchanged at 8 AM and at 9 AM. The cervix was 90% effaced. A thin rim of cervix could be felt by the examiner.

Comment

The diagnosis is an arrest of dilatation in the active phase. Until rotation takes place this cervical rim may persist and should not be a surprise. Had the patient progressed from 8 cm to full dilation with *slow* progression, some obstetricians would have called this the decelerative phase of normal labor.

If progress in active labor stops, usually after 1 hour, think of interventions. In general, think in terms of *all* possible interventions. In the active phase there are seven possible therapeutic interventions—patience, ambulation, analgesia, regional block, ROM, oxytocin, cesarean—and during the second stage of labor forceps and vacuum extraction may be added to the list.

DESCENT AND THE DECELERATIVE PHASE

Descent has not been commented on in most of the earlier discussions; it is more likely that descent will begin as rotation, flexion, and adaptation of the vertex to the pelvis takes place.

If descent is less than 1 cm per hour *after it has started* (ie, it starts and then stops), then it may be labeled as a prolongation or an arrest of descent. The diagnosis of descent arrest should only be made during the second stage of labor. Usually some descent may take place late in active phase or during second stage of labor. A high vertex (station −4 or −5) does not test pelvic capacity until descent begins. The clinician cannot easily predict labor outcome without waiting an adequate time to establish if the pelvis can accommodate the vertex.

PRIMARY AND SECONDARY ARRESTS

The problem of whether an arrest of dilatation is primary or secondary adds little to management plans. Similar statements may be made for arrest of descent. If the process is seen to start and then it stops, it can be called a secondary arrest. The arrest is known to be present because the patient has been examined at two points in time and change was found. For simplicity the terms primary or secondary are not used.

Protractions of Cervical Dilatation

Nullipara:	Less than 1.2 cm for longer than 1 h
Multipara:	Less than 1.5 cm for longer than 1 h

In an earlier study done at Cleveland Metropolitan General Hospital, protraction of active phase dilation was the most frequently occurring dysfunctional labor pattern. Prolonged decelerative phase was the least frequent diagnosis.[3]

For management, protractions should be looked upon as being similar to arrests. The protraction is only a matter of degree and is less easily recognized. The same interventions as those used for treatment of arrests should be applied. Protractions usually have the same etiologies as arrests of labor.

FORMAT FOR ANALYZING AND TREATING ABNORMALITIES

Chart notes, as discussed for latent phase labor, should include a description of the patient's history (if this is the first note rather than a progress note) and management plans. Active phase diagnosis and treatments are introduced again as terms, not to suggest some new methods for patient care, but rather as part of an orderly process. Document what has occurred. Think of what may be done. Consider all patient care options and intervene. This process should be described in the chart note.

Describe the Labor. A note is usually made at the first patient contact during labor. Thus, if the patient has already been admitted and examined, begin at point number 4 below.

1. Include a brief statement about relevant maternal or fetal background factors, one general medical history, and one antepartum course. This should be the first note in the admitting obstetrical record.
2. Is the patient in active labor? After two examinations there should be a note in the patient's chart describing her progress and answering this question.
3. List the intrapartal clinical factors which are important, including cervical dilatation, station, and vertex position.
4. Conclude with a brief description of labor thus far. The interval note is written in the patient's chart. In contrast to latent phase labor when it may not have been possible to describe the observed labor course, in active phase labor there is a labor course to review. The orderly documenting of this information helps to clarify the clinician's thinking during the long hours of labor. Years later the note may be helpful for review purposes.

THERAPEUTIC INTERVENTIONS

Therapeutic interventions move from the simple to the complex. *All* interventions should be considered prior to writing patient orders. Patience and ambulation (or position change) are included as therapeutic interventions because they are methods of labor treatment. The cesarean, vacuum extractor, and forceps interventions are placed last on this list as they are to be used after other measures have failed.

1. Patience
2. Ambulation (and position change)
3. Medication (analgesia)
4. Regional block
5. Oxytocin stimulation
6. Membrane rupture
7. Forceps/vacuum
8. Cesarean

EXAMPLES OF ACTIVE PHASE LABOR ABNORMALITIES

The chart notes should be similar to the notes describing the diagnostic evaluation in cases of active phase labor abnormalities. In the examples, the therapeutic sequences, when possible, are presented as flow diagrams with two possible outcomes. The interventions may not always be as sequential as presented in the list; several may take place at the same time. Judgment for a therapeutic intervention in these examples may differ among individual physicians evaluating the same case. Several interventions may be acceptable. Clinical care involves judgment; the evaluation is subjective, altered by recent experience and often differing when comparisons between clinicians are made. The different physician responses to the same clinical experience suggest that there are usually several options for patient care.

EXAMPLE OF DIAGNOSIS AND TREATMENT OF PROTRACTION AND ARREST OF CERVICAL DILATATION (Figure 9.2)

A 28-year-old nullipara with a normal antepartum history stated that her contractions began 4 hours prior to admission. She was observed in the hospital between 2 PM and 5 PM with progress from 5 to 6 cm of cervix dilatation, 80% effaced, and with the vertex OA at station −3. Her membranes were intact. A 3700-g fetus was estimated. The maternal history was unremarkable. The patient stated that she had not slept well for the past 2 days and was extremely tired. It was apparent she was not tolerating her contractions well. The electronic monitor displayed contractions, each 3 to 4 minutes, with normal heart rate information.

Diagnosis Chart Note

This previously normal patient has a protraction of the active phase as documented by slow dilatation of cervix (1 cm in 3 hours). Although contractions have been moderate, little progress has been made.

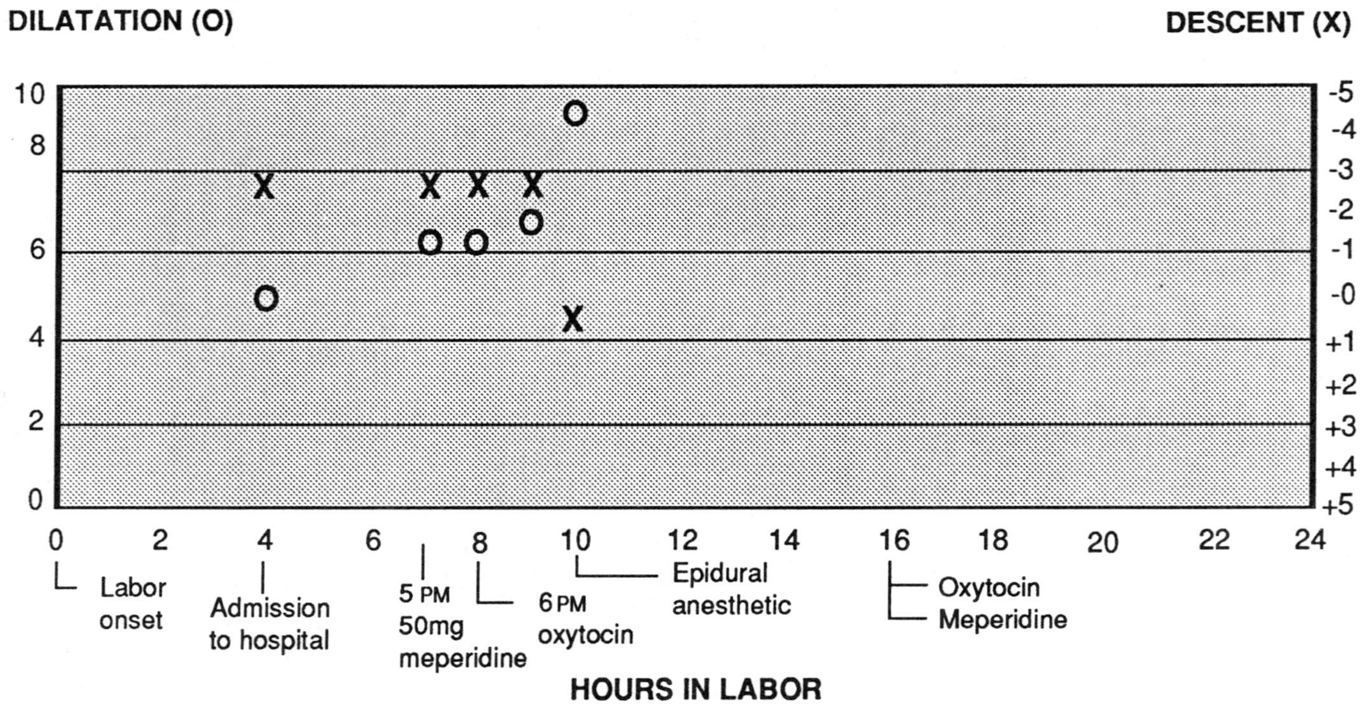
DILATATION (O)
DESCENT (X)
10
8
6
4
2
0
-5
-4
-3
-2
-1
-0
+1
+2
+3
+4
+5
0
2
4
6
8
10
12
14
16
18
20
22
24
Labor onset
Admission to hospital
5 PM 50mg meperidine
6 PM oxytocin
Epidural anesthetic
Oxytocin
Meperidine
HOURS IN LABOR

FIGURE 9.2

5 cm 2 PM

6 cm 5 PM

Protraction of active phase

Therapeutic Choices

1. *Patience:* Waiting longer is probably not a good idea without other support (medication for pain or rest).
2. *Ambulation:* This choice is similar to the patience option. The patient will not walk easily in her present tired, anxious, and painful state.
3. *Medications*
4. *Regional block:* A choice is present here. Meperidine is acceptable. About 50 mg intravenously in a normal size patient would be used. Epidural anesthesia may also be helpful. However, because the uterine forces may be part of the problem, also consider oxytocin augmentation of labor.
5. *Stimulation* (oxytocin): As noted in point number 4 above, oxytocin use is highest on the list of choices to be used in conjunction with some form of pain relief. Medication in a tired patient may lead to 3 to 4 hours of rest with little progress unless oxytocin is also used. At other times pain relief may rapidly increase labor progress.
6. *Membranes:* Many obstetricians would perform artificial rupture of membranes (AROM) as a treatment to improve labor. If oxytocin were used, even more clinicians would rupture the membranes to facilitate internal electronic monitoring. If it is believed that the vertex will not be well applied to the cervix after AROM, membrane rupture should be delayed. In addition, it is not mandatory to perform internal monitoring when using oxytocin if the external monitoring data is acceptable in quality, but it is mandatory to monitor. The information must be technically readable.
7. *Mechanical* (forceps/vacuum): This is not an acceptable intervention at this time.
8. *Cesarean:* This is not an acceptable intervention at this time.

The Labor Continues

50 mg meperidine given and AROM performed

6 cm 5 PM

An arrest is present

6 cm 6 PM

New interventions should be considered because there was no change. The arrest of labor in active phase warrants further treatment.

Oxytocin used to augment arrested labor	6 cm 6 PM
	↓
	7 cm 7 PM

Comment

In the absence of progress, consider problems such as fetal size or position (perhaps the examination of vertex OA position was incorrect). This patient is proceeding in labor like an OP. However, since some progress has occurred (from 6 to 7 cm) the plan is to keep the patient comfortable and continue treatment.

Oxytocin continues Epidural added for pain relief	7 cm 7 PM
	↓
	9 cm 8 PM station 0

Comment

The patient is near the end of active phase. A decelerative phase may follow. The new progress appears acceptable. *Patience* is now added to the clinical routine. As long as progress continues and no indicators of fetal distress are observed, this slow labor, despite the fact that abnormalities (protraction and arrest) have been present, will end in a vaginal birth.

The therapeutic interventions in this case have been:

1. Patience
2. Medication (meperidine, epidural)
3. Stimulation

EXAMPLE OF EARLY INTERVENTION IN QUESTIONABLE LABOR (Figure 9.3)

A 39-year-old G3 P2 mother at 41 weeks of gestation has had a normal antepartum history. Labor contractions began 4 hours ago. On admission to the hospital at 1 AM, the patient was noted to have a term sized fetus, with intact membranes, vertex

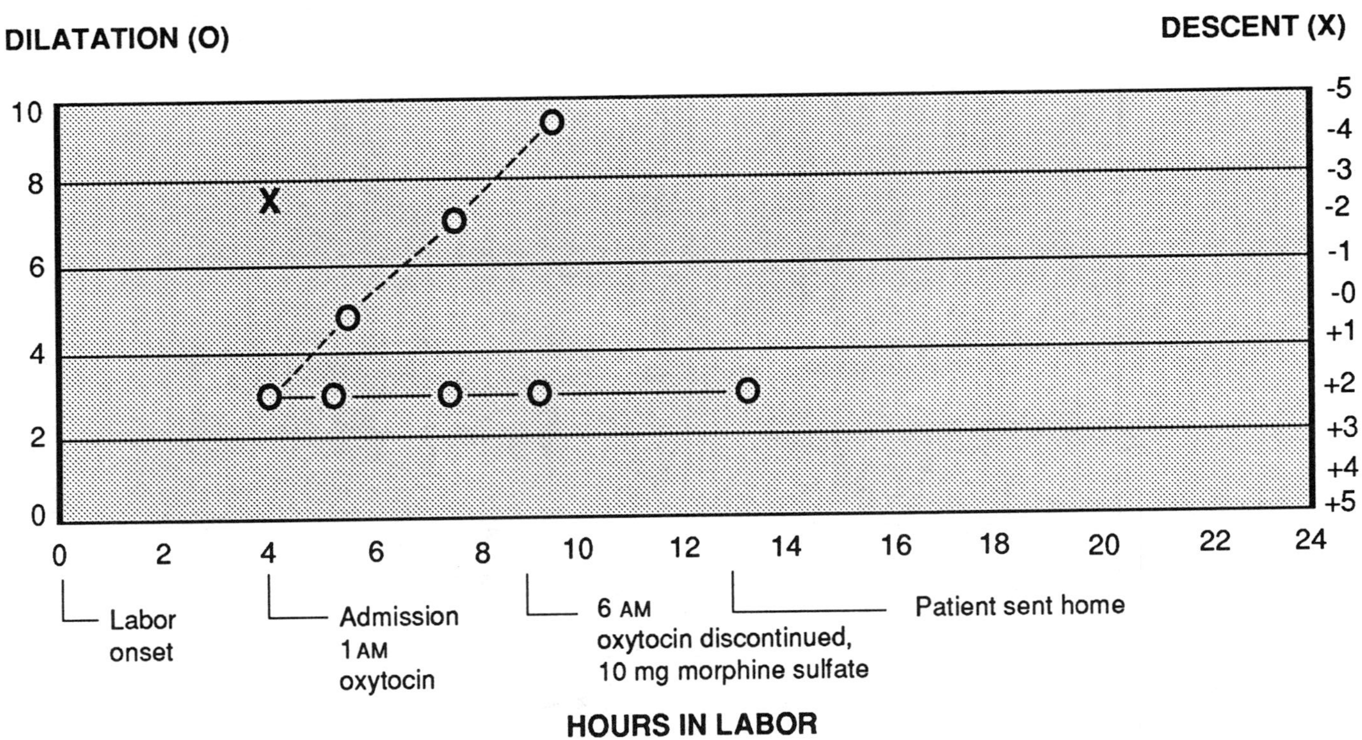
DILATATION (O)
DESCENT (X)
10
8
6
4
2
0
-5
-4
-3
-2
-1
-0
+1
+2
+3
+4
+5
0
2
4
6
8
10
12
14
16
18
20
22
24
Labor onset
Admission
1 AM
oxytocin
6 AM
oxytocin discontinued,
10 mg morphine sulfate
Patient sent home
HOURS IN LABOR

FIGURE 9.3

OP at station −3 cervix 3 cm dilated, 80% effaced, with painful contractions every 7 to 12 minutes.

Diagnostic Chart Note

In the presence of normal antenatal history there is no unusual fetal risk. It is uncertain as to whether the patient is in the latent phase of labor. However, because the patient is at term and the cervix appears to be inducible, an induction will be attempted in order to observe the fetal and maternal responses. The membranes will not be ruptured unless there is an indication for this.

Comment

Maternal age at term in a healthy mother adds no fetal risk during labor. In the office, and without contractions, many clinicians might consider an induction or would suggest that the patient remain at home. In the labor room, in the presence of painful contractions, many clinicians would modify that approach. Despite the factual statement about no increased risk at age 39, inevitably the clinician is influenced by this fact. At 41 weeks of gestation and a ripe inducible cervix, induction of labor at the next convenient time (ie, early the next day) warrants consideration.

Therapeutic Choices

1. *Patience:* This is a possibility and acceptable; other obstetricians may choose to intervene more aggressively.
2. *Ambulation:* Same as number 1.
3. *Medication:*
4. *Regional block:* This is a possibility. However, the patient did not appear tired. Rarely use seconal in the presence of pain. Meperidine analgesia may be considered for this patient. Epidural analgesia would not be considered this early unless the patient's reaction to pain was extremely unusual. In general, try to avoid medication early in labor or until labor is well established. Occasionally use medication for pain relief or anxiety relief at any stage of labor.
5. *Oxytocin:* In this case, the clinician chose to stimulate the patient. However, the obstetrician did not commit herself irrevocably to complete the labor as the membranes were not ruptured. If oxytocin therapy did result in cervical dilatation, the clinician could turn off the oxytocin and even send the patient home.
6. *Membranes:* Many clinicians would choose to rupture membranes at the time of induction. Some benefit is gained from looking for meconium in the amniotic fluid. Try not to rupture membranes unless there are reasons to persist with the induction. If problems in the technique of monitoring arise or fetal distress is questioned, rupture the membranes, insert a pressure catheter, and attach a scalp lead.
7. *Forceps/vacuum:* This is not considered at this time.
8. *Cesarean:* This is not considered at this time.

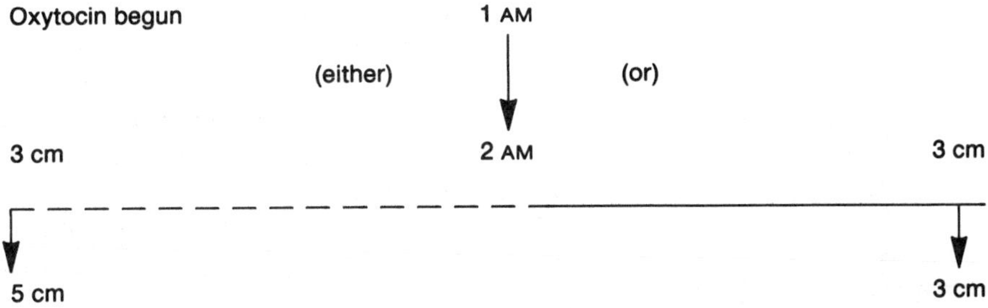

If the cervix had dilated to 5 cm the induction would have been continued.

If the cervix had remained 3 cm dilated, continuing the induction for several additional hours would be considered (Figure 9.3).

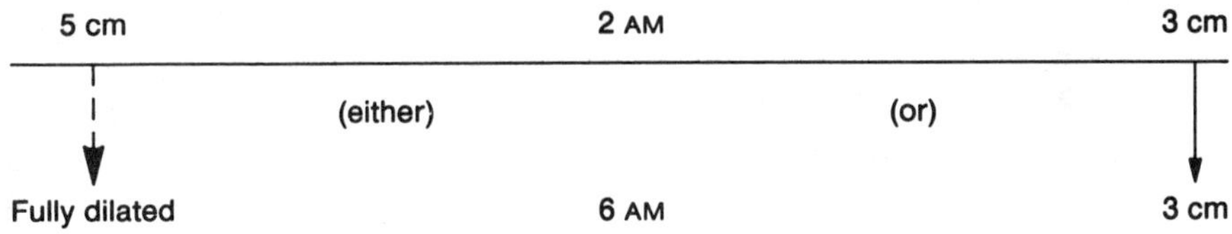

If the cervix becomes fully dilated, the patient is managed as a normal labor, and vaginal delivery is anticipated in the next several hours.

In the alternate situation, with no progress at 3 cm, in the absence of fetal heart rate abnormalities, stop the oxytocin, medicate, and rest the patient, or even send the patient home after the effects of oxytocin have stopped. This decision is predicated on the condition of the patient, including her fatigue, contractions, stress, and personal desires.

History

At 3 cm oxytocin was discontinued and the patient was rested with 10 mg morphine for 4 hours. She awoke with an unchanged cervix and irregular contractions.

Intervention

There is still choice. If induction is started now, look for a long labor. Consider sending this patient home, see her in 2 to 3 days, check the cervix, and await labor. The fetal heart monitoring was reassuring.

FETAL DISTRESS DURING ACTIVE OR SECOND STAGE LABOR

Up to this point active phase labor problems have been considered in the absence of fetal distress. The diagnosis of fetal distress all too frequently appears as a secondary diagnosis when decisions for interventions such as cesareans are made. In reviewing charts of cases such as these, linkage of the diagnoses "failure to progress in labor and fetal distress" occurs too frequently to be acceptable. It appears that the heart rate monitor may provide too easy an excuse to complete the labor. A "little dystocia" and a "possibility of fetal distress" are equivalent to a single correct diagnosis of either dystocia or fetal distress. To be prudent, always consider the possibility of dystocia producing fetal distress. The increased frequency of "failure to progress in labor" and "possible fetal distress" leading to a cesarean cannot be explained.[4,5]

If fetal distress is suspected because of a change in fetal heart beat-to-beat variability, or the observation of occasional variable decelerations (which are common in many labors and are not generally risk factors), obtain better information. Fetal scalp blood examinations are helpful. Between 1975 and 1984, one of the two major reasons for the yearly increase in cesarean birthrates was the increased use of the diagnosis of fetal distress.[5] It is unlikely that obstetricians have learned better methods for identifying fetal distress. Fetal concerns cannot be ignored. In a difficult labor close attention must be paid to all labor events. The diagnosis of dystocia and fetal distress are defined. They should be used accurately when intervention takes place during a difficult labor.

SUMMARY

1. Active phase labor pathology or poor progress is not indicative of fetal damage.
2. A proper chart note should document the labor diagnosis by describing the patient's progress in labor, whether fetal or maternal risk is present, and the anticipated course of the labor.
3. In the chart note, all therapeutic interventions and the reasons for continuing, adding, or changing the patient care plan should be listed.
4. In the absence of obvious maternal or fetal risk factors, there will often be several clinical choices. Management choices will differ among clinicians even when considering the same case. There are few absolutes in clinical care.

REFERENCES

1. Peisner DB, Rosen MG: The latent phase of labor in normal patients: a reassessment. Obstet Gynecol 1985;66:644–648.
2. Peisner D, Rosen MG: Transition from latent to active phase labor. Obstet Gynecol 1986;68:448–451.

3. Sokol RJ, Stojkof J, Chik L, Rosen MG: Normal and abnormal labor progress: I. A quantitative assessment and survey of the literature. J Reprod Med 1977;18:47–53.
4. Rosen, MG: Dystocia, arrest disorders and infant brain damage. Obstet Gynecol 1989;74 (in press).
5. Shiono PH, McNellis D, Rhoads GG: Reasons for the rising cesarean delivery rates: 1978–1984. Obstet Gynecol 1987;69:696–700.

Chapter 10

Dystocia
The Pathology of Labor

OVERVIEW

Previous chapters reviewed the organization of patient care, described neurologic morbidity with respect to labor, defined terminology for the labor stages, and presented treatment programs for abnormal labor patterns. In general all terms and definitions conform to the Friedman nomenclature, which allows for better communication. Use of well-defined terms allows the clinician to intervene in a more orderly and prompt manner when labor is not progressive. In this chapter on pathology of labor, which is very broadly defined, dystocia is presented and placed into the dictionary of terms.

The term dystocia and words such as "cephalopelvic disproportion" (CDP) or "failure to progress" are frequently used in obstetrical diagnoses. They will be reviewed in attempt to remove them from the readers' glossary of terms. These terms are too vague and have different meanings to each investigator.

Howard Taylor, writing in the foreword of Moloy's monograph[1] on pelvic measurements stated that "cephalopelvic disproportion is the chief cause of difficult labor, and difficult labor is still the most important problem in obstetrics." Although 35 years have elapsed since that statement was made, it is still correct today. The term cephalopelvic disproportion, with all of its descriptive vagaries, encompasses a treatment problem responsible for about one third of the primary cesareans performed in the United States.[2] It is difficult to believe that in an era of less crippling illnesses such as poliomyelitis, less bony pelvic distortion due to rickets or scurvy, improved treatment of trauma, and better nutrition, the female pelvic appears less adequate to accommodate vaginal delivery. Yet, the use of dystocia as a diagnosis made by obstetricians continues to be a major treatment problem.[2,3]

OBJECTIVES

At the conclusion of this chapter, the clinician should be able to:

1. Understand the meaning of dystocia with respect to success in vaginal birth
2. Accept the Friedman classification as an adjunct to patient care
3. Describe dystocia in a chart note in terminology which will allow peer review of labor progress
4. Discard the use of terms such as failure to progress, dystocia, and cephalopelvic disproportion in chart notes as indicators for treatment

DYSTOCIA AND BRAIN DAMAGE

The diagnosis of difficult labor should be described in terms of protractions or arrests in the active phase, and in the second stage, as arrests of descent of the vertex. These diagnoses are always made retrospectively, after labor difficulty has become evident, and the fetus already has experienced a portion of labor. The obstetrician is not clairvoyant and should rarely use a labor diagnosis to justify terminating labor in latent phase or before labor upset.

There is data from the mid-1970s which concludes that alteration in birth route as a treatment for dystocia does not alter the incidence of brain damage.[4,5] Note that this more recent evaluation is not the description of dystocia perceived as a neglected labor nor as a traumatic delivery, which was commonly seen in the patient care of previous eras. Today, while the sun may rise on a single labor, it rarely rises twice on a woman in labor.

In a review by Bottoms et al[4] from Cleveland Metropolitan General Hospital, dystocia, defined by protractions and arrests, was not associated with evidence of neurologic morbidity during the neonatal period. The same infant population was reviewed in a follow-up after 2 years of age, or when major neurologic morbidity was first documented.[5] Obstetrical treatments, such as the use of oxytocin, forceps, or cesareans, which were used as interventions in these difficult labors, were studied for their relationship to major brain damage.

The use of oxytocin was not associated with increased infant brain damage when compared with neonates born after similar problem labors delivered without oxytocin.[5] In this particular patient care environment oxytocin use was carefully controlled. Cesareans were rarely performed before a trial of oxytocin was instituted. The usual practice was to start oxytocin and then to anticipate progress within 1 hour, and usually to desist within 3 hours in the absence of progress during active phase or second stage labor. In the Cleveland study, whether delivered by cesarean, low forceps, or midforceps, infant neurologic outcome remained the same. Forceps use in the population was uncommon.

It cannot be stated that dystocia is harmless as the study did not compare dystocia to normal labors. Prospectively, there is no way of avoiding dystocia before it occurs. The available treatment regimens described here are acceptable on the basis of known infant outcome.

In summary, brain damage is not changed by changing birth route in dystocia patients. The variate here is that good judgment is applied in labor management. Intervene if progress does not take place as expected. Heroics or the difficult forceps after the difficult labors are not acceptable.

DYSTOCIA AND REPEAT CESAREANS

Evidence of the inability of clinicians to define what dystocia really is may be found in the studies of vaginal birth after a cesarean for dystocia. More than one half of the patients who have had a trial of labor following a cesarean for dystocia delivered vaginally, and with larger neonates.[6] Some of the responsibility for the outcome of the primary cesarean for dystocia must rest with the obstetrician's judgment of allowing, or not allowing, for an adequate trial of labor. Some difference in outcomes in the following pregnancy include better fetal adaptation to the maternal pelvis. Fetal size apparently is not the problem. Understanding the outcome of labor and birth with respect to clinical pelvimetry and fetal size, mechanical forces of labor, and behavioral influences affecting labor, is at best an inexact science. A diagnosis of dystocia for a previous cesarean should not exclude a trial of labor in the following pregnancy.

CRITERIA FOR DEFINING DYSTOCIA

As noted in Table 10.1, in the past innumerable terms have been used to describe labor. In this text labor is described in terms of latent, active, and second stages, and the Friedman criteria, with minimal modifications, are used. If clinicians use a uniform language and similar definitions such as those listed in Table 10.2, outcomes between different obstetricians acting

TABLE 10.1 Inappropriate Terms for Describing Abnormal Labor

Dystocia
Cephalopelvic disproportion
Failure to progress in labor
Failure of forces in labor
Pelvic contracture
Excessive size fetus

TABLE 10.2 Labor Diagnosis[a]

Term	Criteria[b]
Prolonged latent phase	Nulliparas > 20 h Multiparas > 14 h
Protracted active phase dilatation	Nulliparas < 1.2 cm/h Multiparas < 1.5 cm/h
Arrest of dilatation	No progress for 2 h
Protracted descent	Nulliparas < 1 cm/h Multiparas < 2 cm/h
Arrest of descent	No progress for > 1 h

[a]Modified after Friedman.
[b]Numbers indicate 95 percentile.

on different risk patients with different patterns of care may be compared and evaluated. This will lead to more consistent guidelines for labor management.

ETIOLOGIES FOR ABNORMAL LABORS

No matter how the clinician tries to determine specific etiologies for abnormal labors, there is a tendency to speak in vague general terms using clinical "feelings" and traditionally worded descriptions. For example, in the most specific of circumstances, with a catheter documenting intrauterine pressure during a contraction, a cervix may not dilate and it will not be known why dilation did not take place. The catheter may document symmetrical contractions with adequate pressure peaks, but if the cervix does not dilate, the labor will not progress despite the normal pictures. For these reasons our treatments of labor protractions or arrests is at best pragmatic, involving a series of intervention trials and successes or failures. As long as the principles applied to the various treatments involve avoidance of increased risk to mother and fetus, it is appropriate to continue the labor.

Abnormalities of women in labor have been described in terms of (1) problems of the birth canal; (2) problems of fetal position, presentation, and size; and (3) problems of the forces of labor. Assessment of these three general categories requires assessment of the two patients involved. A vaginal examination, ultrasonography, or viewing contractions portrayed by an electronic monitor, when used alone is inadequate clinical care. Taken in the context of the entire patient picture, tests and evaluations are helpful; they assist the clinician in reaching a diagnosis.

ASSESSING THE MOTHER

Maternal Stature

The female pelvis is only part of the patient's complete physical picture. Maternal height may have an association with pelvic size. The very short or disproportionately built patient may foreshadow problems during labor because of pelvic size. However, for the individual patient, the predictive value of the data about maternal height is vague at best.

The very obese patient may have problems of soft tissue dystocia. These women do have a higher incidence of larger babies.[7] Despite the risks, most obese patients deliver large babies at term without difficulty. Maternal stature alerts the clinician to suspect a potential for a problem, but at best the actual risk for the problem will be quite small. Similarly, the vaginal birth risks may be balanced against maternal anesthetic risk and postoperative morbidity, all of which are increased in association with morbidity.

Measurements of the Birth Canal

Clinical measurements of the pelvis have already been described in Chapter 3. They are best performed early in pregnancy before the fetal vertex is in the pelvis. During labor, because of fetal position, poor pelvic muscle relaxation, or maternal discomfort, pelvic measurements may be difficult to perform. As an example, most pelvic sidewalls feel convergent when examined during labor.

Two measurements may be helpful during labor.

1. *The diagonal conjugate* is too short if less than 11.5 cm, and may foreshadow a problem labor in which the vertex may not engage. This measurement is less easily made during labor, as it is painful to perform and the vertex may be in the way.

2. *The prominence of the ischial spines* may help document the size of the midpelvis. If the vertex is at or near the ischial spines, the inlet usually has been traversed, the vertex is engaged, and thus a size mismatch between pelvis and fetal head should be no problem. In contrast, prominent ischial spines may foreshadow problems in vertex rotation and descent in the midpelvis. Even in the presence of suspected prominent ischial spines and a short diagonal conjugate, dilation of the cervix should take place. The labor will declare itself if given adequate time. The cervix should dilate even if descent cannot be completed. If, in the presence of a small pelvis, membranes are ruptured, the membranes as a dilating wedge will no longer be able to assist in the cervical dilatation. If the vertex does not descend it may not be applied to the cervix, and once again dilatation will become a problem as it may not be seen.

The simplified description of intrapartum pelvic assessment does not infer that the shape, position, and curve of the sacrum; the size of the sacrosciatic notch (1 to 3 finger breadths); and the splay of the side walls of the pelvis (convergent, straight, or divergent) are not helpful. It is just that during labor these measurements are difficult to perform. As observed in teaching exercises with residents, or by the questions asked at residency and specialty examinations, it is apparent that there is a widespread lack of knowledge of pelvic architecture and of the measurements of the pelvis.

Some clinicians argue that attempting to measure or assess the clinical pelvis is a waste of time. In this text it is still presented as useful information. First, picture the three-dimensional shape of the birth canal; this assists in thinking in terms of why a vertex does not rotate or descend. There is a distance that must be traversed and adapted to for the passage to take place.

EXAMPLE

Some vertex presentations deliver occiput posterior because of fetal size and maternal pelvic shape. The occiput posterior birth of an average size baby will demonstrate a long molded vertex, far different from the occiput anterior vertex birth. This "shaping" of the head had to take place or the fetal diameters would not allow adaptation and descent to take place.

Knowledge of pelvic shape allows the clinician to think about birth mechanisms in terms of fetal and pelvic sizes and shapes. The pelvis as a birth canal becomes more easily visible.

EXAMPLE

If forceps are to be applied, the clinician understands that there is a curve to the sacrum along which the pelvic curve of the forceps blade must be guided. Similarly, ischial spines impinge on the passageway and the forceps application must be guided by these points. In the presence of prominent ischial spines, if rotation is to be performed, it should take place above or below the spines which are preventing spontaneous vertex rotation.

The vertex must flex and descend beneath the symphysis pubis before the vertex can be extended over the perineum. Lack of understanding as to where to flex the vertex under the symphysis may lead to increased pressure on the vertex. Early vertex extension leads to the use of more traction force and potential trauma.

PELVIS AND FORCEPS TRACTION

When applying traction, understanding the three-dimensional qualities of the birth canal allows application of traction in a lower direction (towards the floor) when the vertex is above the perineum, and in a more horizontal direction as the vertex first flexes below the symphysis pubis and then extends after the occiput has passed under the symphysis. The use of pelvimetry provides a clinical concept of how birth may take place and how forceps traction may be used.

USE OF X-RAY PELVIMETRY AND TOMOGRAPHY PRIOR TO OR DURING LABOR

X-ray pelvimetry is no longer a useful routine and is not a required measurement for vertex births. In the preface to his monograph on pelvimetry, Thoms[8] noted that all patients on the University Service of the Grace New Haven Hospital during the previous 25 years had undergone x-ray measurements. That day is long since gone. Today use of x-ray pelvimetry is infrequent. Radiologists or radiology technicians have sufficient training to obtain adequate films for study. No recent studies documenting the usefulness of x-ray pelvimetry have been performed.

The evaluation of computerized tomography is also ill-defined. The technique may hold more promise for precise pelvic measurements. Before computer average tomography pelvimetry is accepted as useful, studies must be performed in a controlled manner demonstrating the prognostic accuracy of the technique.

Despite the above statements, all too often the radiologic demonstration of a below-average-size pelvis (still normal, not contracted, but just below average) is equated with too small a pelvis and is used as a reason for terminating labor (or avoiding it in the first place). A small pelvis is frequently diagnosed in the presence of breech presentation. The reported findings may represent an obstetrical bias against the vaginal delivery.

ASSESSING THE FETUS: FETAL SIZE, FETAL ABNORMALITIES

Fetal bony abnormalities, such as hydrocephalus or abnormal growths or tumors, speak for themselves. However, fetal size, large or small, is not usually an indicator for avoiding labor. Arguments have been made for arbitrarily setting limits for vaginal birth at 4500 g. No clear end point is available. Rather, the passenger and the pelvis need to be assessed.

In the presence of a large fetus be wary of labors which do not progress easily and without stimulation. A vertex not engaged at labor onset is a usual finding with a large size fetus. However, a greater concern is that in labor, a large vertex followed by larger shoulders engages the vertex; the vertex then delivers, but shoulder dystocia is not predictable. While shoulder dystocia has a higher incidence in large fetuses, the majority of shoulder problems take place in normal size fetuses. In general, when ultrasonography data predicts the birth of a larger than 4000-g fetus,[9] the incidence of shoulder dystocia will rise. This should not be an excuse to avoid a trial of labor; however, this information should caution the clinician to limit interventions such as oxytocin or forceps. The delivery of the 4000-g fetus vaginally is acceptable and usual. Become more concerned about disproportion between fetal vertex and shoulders when estimates of fetal weight exceed 4500 g. Arbitrary fetal size limits are not suggested.

EXAMPLE

A large mother with a history of having delivered fetuses between 4000 and 4500 g is evaluated differently than an expected large fetus in a short nulliparous mother.

Comment

There is no rule or standard beyond which size estimates of the vertex should be delivered by cesarean. Certainly in the 4000- to 4500-g range caution and preparation for the birth is in order. Anticipating a large fetus, the obstetrician should prepare for the birth in a delivery room environment and with anesthetic support available rather than in a birthing environment where emergency support will be limited.

ULTRASONOGRAPHY TO DETERMINE FETAL SIZE

With the use of ultrasonography, the documentation of fetal weight and size is quite helpful. It must be understood that at the extremes of fetal size there is less accuracy in the estimations. As noted in the preceding section, the use of a cesarean in fetuses between 9 lb (4000 g) and 10 lb (4500 g) is not mandated. Certainly more aggressive intervention, such as oxytocin or forceps use, should be considered with extreme caution. If the labor is proceeding well, allow it to proceed. If progress is poor or arrested, the labor-ending decisions are reached more easily. For the rare patient with expected fetal weight beyond 10 lb, or 4500 g, look for antecedent medical problems, such as diabetes or maternal obesity. The clinician who uses a cesarean without a trial of labor in the 4500-g fetus has not infrequently found that clinical and ultrasonographic predictions of fetal size did not correlate with the neonatal weight. Many times the fetus estimated to weigh over 4500 g results in a 4100-g neonate. In general, await labor onset; then a judgment which may vary between clinicians is made. If the vertex descends and labor is proceeding well, deliver the patient vaginally. In contrast, with a high vertex at labor onset and slow progress, move promptly to a cesarean.

FETAL MECHANICS

The way a fetus is moved through the pelvis during labor is poorly understood and rarely even thought of. Labor necessitates adaptation of the fetal body and head to the maternal pelvis. The teaching of labor mechanics, for example, that in the vertex presentation there is internal rotation, descent, and flexion, and, with birth, there is vertex extension and external rotation, is a neglected part of clinical care education.

It may be helpful if the clinician thinks in terms of the following patterns. If the vertex is in the occiput posterior or transverse position, it is generally poorly flexed. The vertex may be deflexed or even extended. The fetus will need to descend and to flex in order to present a smaller diameter for birth, and labor will take more time.

An extended vertex may deliver vaginally if it extends or rotates. A face may deliver vaginally if it engages and rotates to a mentum anterior position. Many face presentations will remain high and will not engage. For example, if the vertex is extended and does not descend, think of a possible brow presentation which is usually undelivered.

When the cervix stops dilating in the active phase, look for an abnormality in fetal mechanics as well as uterine forces. Frequently, the cervix will not dilate completely if the vertex remains high and unengaged in the pelvis. Rotation to an anterior position may not occur. In contrast, at the level of station +3 within the pelvis, the vertex in posterior position may deliver in that position. Because the occiput posterior diameters are larger than the occiput anterior diameters, far more effort is needed in this fetal situation and increased vertex molding and longer second stage labors are anticipated.

Similar to problems of flexion and rotation, keep in mind lateral flexion or *asynclitism* (flexion to the side). These fetal mechanical problems create labor difficulties involving more pressure, more molding, and more time.

Problems which relate to the mechanics of labor generally do not occur in a single fetal diameter. Generally, a vertex left occiput transverse is also asynclitic. These situations lead to more difficult labors associated with protractions and arrests of dilatation and descent. The Friedman system allows documentation of the problem but does not give the reasons for the problems. Treatment individualized to the clinical problem may include position change, ambulation, oxytocin, regional anesthesia, or combinations of these therapeutic measures.

MOLDING OF THE VERTEX

It is not easily explained as to why some patients still in latent phase labor and at high pelvic stations already present with caput and molding of the vertex. At times, even overriding of the parietal bones at the sagittal suture may be seen with a vertex at relatively high stations of the pelvis. In contrast, note some patients with relatively short latent and active phases, and with a fully dilated cervix, show little caput or molding of the vertex. The unmolded fetal vertex may need more time in second stage of labor to acquire the molding before the vertex will deliver. Generally, both caput and molding will correlate with fetal size and labor length.

In today's less aggressive vaginal birth environment, the occurrence of a dural sinus laceration secondary to excessive vertex molding, following a too long labor or a difficult forceps, should be rare. Cohen's data[10] on second stage labor shows that in the second stage, time and patience beyond the 1- and 2-hour limits is acceptable. Thus, 3 or perhaps 4 hours of watchful waiting in the absence of fetal distress and in the presence of continuing progress is acceptable. Judgment and caution are also included in this plan. When descent is slow but continues, and the second stage lengthens, observation of continuing descent overtime is appropriate. Intervention with midforceps should be infrequent as these labors foreshadow difficult instrument deliveries.

ASSESSING THE UTERINE FORCES

Correlating Contractions with Progress

A protraction or an arrest of labor may be seen either in the presence of less frequent or less strong uterine contractions, or both. In a protraction or arrest of labor one expects to see an analog of this pattern on the electronic monitoring record. In contrast, protractions or arrests may also occur even in the presence of good contractions, which appear as bell-shaped curves associated with adequate intrauterine pressure levels and with contractions each 2 to 3 minutes. This is not what is expected. The monitoring pictures and the patient's progress do not always coincide. Do not stimulate a labor in which progress is good but the monitor is not displaying the expected patterns. Similarly, stimulate a labor that is not progressing but in which the in utero pressure pattern is as perfect as the expected contraction picture.

EXAMPLE

Contractions began 4 hours prior to admission in a G3 P2 at term patient with normal antepartum and past history. She was admitted at 5 cm dilatation, vertex at station −2, 80% cervical effacement, and spontaneous rupture of membranes about 1 hour before (Figure 10.1). An average size fetus was expected. In the hospital during the next 2 hours, despite the presence of apparently adequate contractions, no progress was seen. Dilatation remained at 4 cm.

The obstetrician chose to medicate the patient with 50 mg of demerol intravenously and begin an oxytocin infusion. One hour later the patient was 8 cm dilated. At this time, an epidural block was administered for pain relief.

Comment

Many intervention choices were acceptable here. At 5 cm the patient is considered —if in labor—in active phase. Without progress for 2 hours it is possible this was not labor, but highly unlikely. The use of oxytocin was acceptable as long as monitoring confirmed absence of fetal placental supply problems. Medication for pain relief was another acceptable treatment alone, or in concert with the oxytocin. Almost all treatment modalities except labor termination were acceptable in this patient.

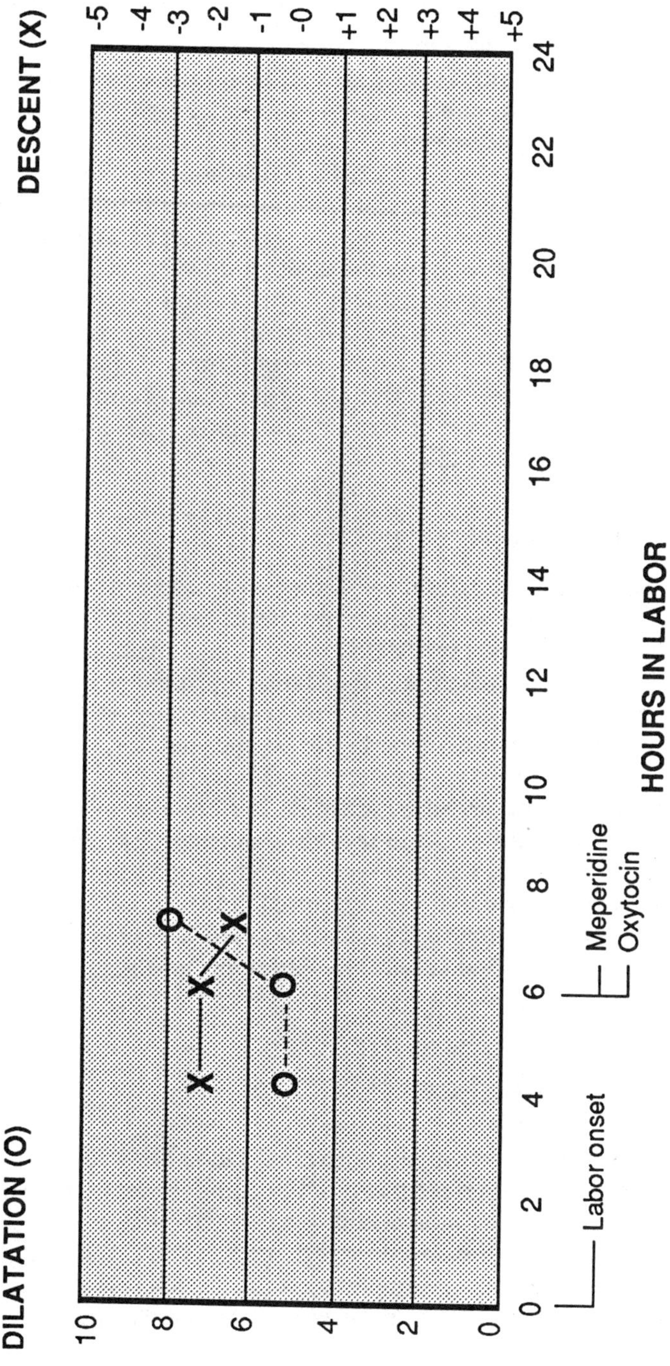
DILATATION (O)
DESCENT (X)
10
8
6
4
2
0
-5
-4
-3
-2
-1
-0
+1
+2
+3
+4
+5
0
2
4
6
8
10
12
14
16
18
20
22
24
Labor onset
Meperidine
Oxytocin
HOURS IN LABOR

FIGURE 10.1

Physiology or Pathophysiology of Contractions and Labor

Transition from the laboratory to the labor bed and from muscle contraction to labor understanding has been slow. It is not understood why labor contractions start and why labor begins. More is known about why and how the uterine smooth muscle contracts. Contractions can be stimulated or stopped. Yet, little is known about the propagation of the contraction throughout the uterus and why electronic monitoring of some contractions produces a skewed curve displayed on the paper tracing, and other contractions produce bell-shaped curves on the recording charts. Little is understood about the contraction pattern or its physiology. It is not understood why the contractions, good or poor, may or may not dilate the cervix. It is almost impossible to assess uterine forces or effectiveness of function accurately between the extremes of no contractions and tetanic contractions. For these reasons the clinician learns to judge labor not upon contractions, but on cervical dilatation.

Criteria for Effective Contractions

The criteria for evaluation of uterine forces is a judgment made at the bedside and in association with clinical progress.

Questions to be asked are: Is progress, as documented by cervical dilatation, taking place? Is there a prolongation of latent phase or a protraction or an arrest present in active or second stage of labor? This information is more meaningful than the shape and frequency of the contraction.

There are fetal questions to be asked in the presence of contraction abnormalities. Is the fetal heart rate recording normal? Specifically, is the tracing without evidence of late decelerations which may indicate uterine flow is being restricted secondary to abnormal contractions?

In summary, the criterion for effective contractions is good progress in labor associated with expected cervical dilatation in the absence of signs of fetal distress.

DYSFUNCTIONAL LABOR

Terms such as dyscoordinate or dysfunctional labor are frequently used and poorly understood. These terms do not adequately define the pathology of the problem and are not useful. The visual picture of frequent contractions with little progress in cervical dilatation is well-known. In the presence of abnormalities of contraction frequency and shape, think in terms of the entire system—labor progress and fetal condition.

When the electronic findings suggest adequate forces are present but the clinical findings show poor progress, the choice of clinical interventions are not clear. Proceed in a trial and observation mode. In these situations consider ambulation in a rested patient and regional block before oxytocin use. However, even in the presence of what appears to be good uterine contractions, careful use of oxytocin may provide a more adequate trial of labor. Close observation and avoidance of any evidence of delayed decelerations or signs of fetal deprivation of supply or distress is needed.

TREATMENT PROGRAM FOR DYSTOCIA: ACTIVE MANAGEMENT PROTOCOL

The active management system proposed by some authors involves graphing labor beginning from the time of entry into the labor suite and early intervention with oxytocin.[11,12] These authors are proponents of a system that does not define latent and active phases of labor. Labor pictured as a straight line is expected to progress with 1 cm/h of cervical dilatation. Oxytocin is used if the patient does not conform to the expected rate of cervical dilatation. Labor, which is generally defined by entry into the labor room, is completed in 10 hours. The second stage ends in 2 hours, usually without forceps and is associated with low cesarean birthrates. These authors[11,12] suggest that uterine rupture resulting from oxytocin use is rare when used in nulliparous patients.

In this active management protocol, monitoring is used to avoid fetal distress. In the original active management protocol, oxytocin as a medical treatment was not used in the multiparous patient for fear of uterine rupture.[10] It was inferred in this treatment plan that poor forces of labor were the problems with most abnormal labors, and cephalopelvic disproportion could be ruled out and avoided by trial of labor. Most multiparas will manage these problems spontaneously without the use of oxytocin. As suggested by Cardozo et al,[13] problems of position, such as rotation (occiput posterior, occiput transverse), deflexion, and descent are secondary to inadequate uterine forces.

In this text, adherence to a protocol of "active labor management" is not urged. However, intervening earlier and more frequently with oxytocin augmentation is an individualized patient care theme. The use of oxytocin in all patients, including multiparous women, is acceptable. It is understood that with increasing parity and uterine size, prudent judgment associated with this treatment mode must be exercised according to the individual patient.

Most clinicians use modifications of this "active labor management" approach. Individualized patient management is offered. Utilize all the potential treatment measures including time, ambulation, membrane rupture, and oxytocin. The Friedman system documents what is happening at any moment in time better than the arbitrary 1 cm/h guideline for dilatation. Admitting patients later in latent phase or active phase labor, and anticipating slow or faster time periods for cervical dilatation and vertex descent, is part of the plan offered in this text.

SUMMARY

1. Neurologic pathology following difficult labors, defined as protractions or arrests, has not decreased with the increased use of cesarean in dystocia.
2. The term dystocia is a vague descriptor for a difficult labor and should be discarded.
3. Terms such as cephalopelvic disproportion, failure of forces, uterine inertia, and dysfunctional labor should no longer be used as labor diagnoses.
4. Labor should be described in terms of latent, active, and second stages with normal or abnormal progress described as protractions or arrests of dilatation or descent.

REFERENCES

1. Moloy HC: Clinical and Roentgenologic Evaluation of the Pelvis in Obstetrics. Philadelphia, London, WB Saunders, 1951 (foreword by HC Taylor, Jr).
2. Shiono PH, McNellis DM, Rhoads CC: Reasons for the rising cesarean delivery rates, 1978–84. Obstet Gynecol 1987;69:696–700.
3. Shiono PH, Fielden JG, McNellis D, et al: Recent trends in cesarean birth and trial of labor rates in the U.S. JAMA 1987;257:494–497.
4. Bottoms SF, Hirsch VJ, Sokol RJ: Medical management of arrest disorders of labor: a current overview. Am J Obstet Gynecol 1987;156:935–939.
5. Rosen MG: Arrest disorders and infant brain damage. Obstet Gynecol 1989;74 (in press).
6. Cesarean Childbirth, publication 82-2067. Bethesda, MD, National Institutes of Health, October 1981, pp 159–239.
7. Gross TL, Sokol RS, King KC: Obesity and pregnancy: risks and outcomes. Obstet Gynecol 1980;56:446–450.
8. Thoms H: Pelvimetry. New York, Paul B. Hoeber, Inc, 1956, p 9.
9. Acker DB, Sachs BP, Friedman EA: Risk factors for shoulder dystocia. Obstet Gynecol 1985;66:762–768.
10. Cohen WR: The influence of the duration of the second stage of labor on perinatal outcome and puerperal morbidity. Obstet Gynecol 1977;49:266–269.
11. O'Driscoll K, Foley M, MacDonald D: Active management of labour as an alternative to cesarean section. Obstet Gynecol 1984;63:485–490.
12. Philpott RH: The recognition of cephalopelvic disproportion. Clin Obstet Gynecol 1982;9:609–624.
13. Cardozo LD, Gibbs DMF, Shedd JW, et al: Predictive value of cervicometric labor patterns in primigravidae. Br J Obstet Gynaecol 1982;89:33–38.

Chapter 11

Forceps

Historical Background and the Debate

OVERVIEW

Almost from the moment forceps were invented, their use—or misuse—was debated. Today, forceps should remain an acceptable choice for the obstetrician. Midforceps may be used. Midforceps use as a group of procedures cannot easily be separated from terms such as difficult or easy midforceps, or even terms such as low midforceps, or low or outlet forceps. If low forceps are used, inevitably midforceps will be used on the occasion in which a strict criteria for the definition of low forceps is not applied. The physician tends to describe forceps as lower in classification because of the opprobrium which often follows the term "mid" associated with forceps.

The term midforceps is too broad. For example, a midforceps performed from station +1 is far more difficult and the maternal and fetal effects must also be different when compared with a midforceps performed at station +3 or +4 in a five-station pelvis.

In this chapter, the evolution of forceps will be reviewed, and the origins of the midforceps debate will be described. Findings relating infant outcome to midforceps use will be presented. Finally, a new series of definitions for forceps classification will be proposed; in this case based on the station the forceps were applied and the position of the vertex. The key principle in this chapter is the use of clinical judgment. There are choices in clinical care and there is no need to return to difficult and traumatic deliveries.

OBJECTIVES

At the conclusion of this chapter, the clinician should understand:

1. The historical origins of the midforceps debate
2. The clinical data leading to the decision for continuing midforceps use

A BRIEF HISTORY OF FORCEPS

Claude Heaton, waxing poetic in the preface to Dennen's classic monograph *Forceps Deliveries*,[1] wrote: "The obstetrical forceps has been described as a noble and beneficent instrument rescuing more lives and cutting short more pains than all other instruments in the professional armamentarium." Heaton described the invention of forceps by Peter Chamberlen, Sr, a French Huguenot refugee who went to England in 1569. At first in secret, the use of forceps became well-known after Edmund Chapman published information on forceps use in 1733.[1] Obviously, not all clinicians were then or remain now as sanguine as Dr. Heaton about the use of these instruments for facilitating birth. Speert,[2] writing more conservatively of obstetrical interventions, presented a negative view: "Nature is the best judge in childbearing in a normal process; nature should be allowed to take its course." To paraphrase Speert, don't rush to use forceps or to intervene. Today this perspective is encouraged.

An even more negative approach to forceps use was reported in a review by Richardson et al, published in 1985.[3] Richardson quoted William Hunter's writing on forceps use in the mid-1700s. "It was a thousand pities (forceps) were invented, where they save one, they murder twenty." In the early 19th century, as a result of changing physician attitudes derived from the early misuse of forceps, they had all but been eliminated.[3] The classic triple tragedy known to all obstetricians exemplified a period of time when forceps use was not advocated. In that episode, fetal death occurred following a protracted labor, followed by Princess Charlotte's death. This was a labor in which forceps use may have saved either of the potential rulers of England. The alternative, the cesarean, would have been mortal for the future queen.[3]

As anesthesia, surgical technology, and understanding of infection advanced, the use of forceps returned. Dr. Joseph Clark, Master of the Rotunda between 1786 and 1793, reported average forceps use in one of 743 births.[3] In 1875, more than 100 years later, Dr. George Johnson, then Master of the Rotunda, reported a remarkably increased forceps rate of one in ten births.[3] Obviously attitudes towards this instrument had changed.

To a large degree, the use of forceps became universal in the 1900s when Delee, in 1921, advocated the prophylactic use of forceps to shorten the second stage of labor. This reflected the 2-hour rule discussed in earlier chapters. By 1951, Dieckman reported that 68% of all births at the Chicago Lying-In Hospital were facilitated with forceps.[3]

Throughout the history of forceps, almost seasonal advocacy or restriction of their use has continued. Duncan Reid[4] encouraged the use of oxytocin, thus leading to a decreased need for forceps use. In 1953, E. Steward Taylor[5] proposed elimination of midforceps because of their marked destructive maternal and fetal effects. In the 1960s, under his stewardship, midforceps were all but eliminated at the University of Colorado in Denver.

Friedman et al[6] suggested that protractions, arrests, and midforceps labors were associated with lower IQs in children at 7 years of age. In contrast to midforceps, low forceps did not show similar outcomes in the study. Friedman and this author have debated this finding publicly. It should be noted that comparable births by cesarean following abnormal labors (the appropriate comparison population) were not studied in the Friedman report.

Today the question remains that if abnormal labor is present, a finding that can only be diagnosed once it is present, how may the patient be delivered? The fetus must be born. Forceps trauma to mother and fetus have been described in many studies. Comparable data of birth route by cesarean in the presence of dystocia randomly substituted for birth route by midforceps is not available.

A second question still facing the clinician is whether the change in birth route, once the labor diagnosis has been made, will alter infant morbidity. To end this review, but not the debate, a report by Kadar and Romero[7] notes that 75% of instrumentally delivered primigravidas delivered heavier babies spontaneously in the next gestation. The authors also note that in the remainder of the studied population, operative delivery was six times greater than in the normal population. This suggests that the original midforceps group will be at risk for later labor difficulties even though three out of four mothers may deliver fetuses spontaneously in the next birth. As noted in vaginal birth after cesarean studies, a second pregnancy usually correlates with a first pregnancy labor experience, and the normal outcomes exceed the problem outcomes.

DATA FROM THE CLEVELAND MIDFORCEPS PROGRAM

To attempt to rationalize this problem—to use or not to use the midforceps—the data from Cleveland Metropolitan General Hospital during the late 1970s and early 1980s was reviewed.[8,9] At that hospital midforceps application was acceptable, but it was urged that midforceps use be performed with an experienced physician present, with caution, and in general at lower (low mid) pelvic stations. The term elective midforceps was not used. There was no "teaching" midforceps use. Midforceps were performed primarily for arrests or protractions in the second stage of labor at midpelvic stations or for fetal distress. The judgment to use midforceps, as taught by the faculty, was to neither "look for trouble" nor to try to demonstrate unusual technical skill. Rather, prior to forceps use, it was up to the physician to judge if, in a patient at a particular pelvic station, forceps use was a safe alternative birth for mother and fetus.

Retrospective studies compared infant outcome between cesarean birth and forceps delivery. The outcome variable sought was major infant brain damage. Data was collected from matched infant chart notes with similar labor diagnoses. The hypothesis was that in the restricted approach to midforceps, their use was not associated with increased risk for mother or infant. This hypothesis could not be disproved. The meaning of "restricted" becomes more apparent when it is noted that the incidence of midforceps use was less than 1% of all births. Forceps applications at stations 0 and +1 were not encouraged, and pelvic station +2 was borderline for decision-making of the five pelvic stations.

The findings documented that there was a significantly higher rate of active phase and second stage labor abnormalities in the midforceps-use group than in the general population. This was understandable since therapeutic interventions, such as patience, sedation, ambulation, position change, membrane rupture, and oxytocin use, were encouraged before considering the "ending" of labor by forceps or cesarean.

Latent phase labor abnormalities were not significantly increased in the midforceps-use group when compared with all other patients, demonstrating once again that terminating a labor in latent phase is generally not an adequate trial for vaginal birth, and that a prolonged latent phase does not predict a difficult active phase or abnormal second stage of labor. No increases in midforceps use in the over 4000-g fetuses was found. Midforceps use in excessive size infants was not encouraged.

Short-term neonatal morbidity, including depressed Apgar scores, seventh nerve palsy, and neonatal seizures, were found to be the same for both midforceps and cesarean birth infants born with the same labor abnormalities. The midforceps group did exhibit a higher incidence of cephalhematomata.

Continuing this study of infants born between 1976 and 1982, through the first 2 years of life, matching the use of forceps for labor abnormality or for fetal distress, no significant differences in infant abnormal neurologic development were found.[9] While these two studies will obviously not end the debate, they at least allow for the generalizations made about midforceps use proposed in Chapter 12.

SUMMARY

1. Midforceps use was more common when cesareans were not an available birth route choice.
2. During the early years of their use, midforceps led to many traumatic injuries to mother and fetus.
3. Changes in technology led to the replacement of difficult midforceps with the cesarean.
4. As safe alternatives to midforceps use became available, efforts to remove forceps from obstetrical therapy returned.
5. Neither prophylactic forceps use during the second stage of labor nor the 2-hour rule arose from data which warranted their application as dogma.
6. In the Cleveland study, selected midforceps use reveals no increase in long-term infant morbidity when compared with cesarean births performed for the same clinical indications.

REFERENCES

1. Dennen EA: Forceps Deliveries. Philadelphia, FA Davis, 1955.
2. Speert H: Obstetrics and Gynecology in America: A History. Baltimore, Waverly Press, 1980, p 38.
3. Richardson DA, Evans M, Cibils L: Midforceps delivery: a critical review. Am J Obstet Gynecol 1983;145:621–632.
4. Reid DE: Treatment of prolonged labor with posterior pituitary extract. Am J Obstet Gynecol 1946;52:719–734.
5. Taylor ES: Can midforceps operations be eliminated. Obstet Gynecol 1953;2:302–307.
6. Friedman EA, Sachtleben MR, Dahrouge D, Neff R: Long-term effects of labor and delivery on offspring: a matched pair analysis. Am J Obstet Gynecol 1984;150:941–945.
7. Kadar N, Romero R: Prognosis for future childbearing after midcavity instrumental deliveries in primigravidas. Obstet Gynecol 1983;62:166–170.
8. Dierker LJ, Rosen MG, Debanne S, Thompson K: The midforceps: maternal and neonatal outcomes. Am J Obstet Gynecol 1985;152:176–183.
9. Dierker LJ, Rosen MG, Thompson K, Linn P: Midforceps—long-term outcome of infants. Am J Obstet Gynecol 1986;154:764–768.

Chapter 12

Forceps
Practical Considerations

OVERVIEW

In Chapter 11, the history of forceps use was reviewed, and the continuing controversy was discussed of whether midforceps should ever be used, and, if used, at what pelvic stations. In this chapter, a classification for forceps use is presented as well as a guide to forceps use. The suggested new classification allows both the operator and the reviewer of the procedure to have a better understanding of what pelvic station the "midforceps" are applied and the degree of difficulty implied from this knowledge. It is suggested that the term midforceps be replaced with this new pelvic station classification.

While this is not a textbook on technique, some technical information is reviewed, including when forceps should be used, the types of forceps suggested for use, and how traction may be better applied. The role of the vacuum extractor is also discussed.

OBJECTIVES

At the conclusion of this chapter, the clinician should be able to:

1. Present definitions for forceps classification
2. Replace terms such as midforceps or low forceps with the new classification based on the pelvic station at which forceps are applied
3. Understand the guidelines for forceps use
4. Discuss basic types of forceps and understand some technical considerations in forceps use

DEFINITIONS AND TERMINOLOGY

Medical and legal implications associated with the term midforceps has led to changes in behavior and has often resulted in incorrect classification of the charted data by the physician. The terms low forceps and midforceps are extremely broad. While the current terminology is presented, the use of a more simple forceps classification—one based on pelvic station and vertex position—is proposed. The term midforceps should be removed from obstetrics because, regardless of the degree of forceps difficulty, it categorically carries with it the long-standing stigma of the debate by physicians as to whether midforceps should ever be used and the implication of trauma connected to the term midforceps.

High forceps are defined as forceps applied when the presenting part, the vertex, is above station 0 as documented by palpating the ischial spines, or when forceps are applied through an incompletely dilated cervix. High forceps are not suggested in safe clinical procedures.

Midforceps are classically defined by the presence of the vertex at or below the ischial spines (station 0 or below) and above the perineum. The perineum is station 5 in a five-station classification of the pelvis or station 3 in a three-station pelvic classification. The cervix must be fully dilated. Rotation may or may not be used. All rotations beyond the oblique, that is left occiput anterior (LOA) or right occiput anterior (ROA), by definition are classified as midforceps.

Recently, the American College of Obstetrics and Gynecology (ACOG) released new terminology redefining these categories which contrasts with the classical definitions. In the new definition ACOG defines midforceps as forceps use from engagement but with the presenting part above S+2 (three pelvic stations).

Low midforceps is a term which is not easily defined. Usually it signifies forceps applied with the vertex at station +3 or +4, and with the cervix fully dilated. Rotation may be performed in this category. Some physicians define midforceps at stations 0 and +1. Low midforceps describes station +2, +3, and +4. These descriptors are still limited in that they do not clearly provide an understanding of forceps difficulty. The ACOG terminology does not have a category of low midforceps.

Low or outlet forceps are terms used interchangeably by some physicians, but not all. The term signifies that the vertex is on the perineum, station +5, and in the occiput anterior (OA) diameter. The vertex should be "crowning" without spreading the labia.

A further point for discussion here is the meaning of the anteroposterior (AP) diameter. Most clinicians include the oblique vertex position (ROA or LOA) within the context of low or outlet forceps. For example, if the vertex is in the occiput transverse (OT) position, application is considered midforceps even if at station +5 because of rotation. In contrast, if the vertex is occiput posterior (OP) and delivered from the OP position by forceps at station +5, but without rotation, it is considered a low or outlet forceps. In summary, all rotations (except the oblique ROA or LOA) are considered as mid at any station.

ACOG has divided the low forceps category into separate sections.[1] Low forceps are defined as being when the leading point of the skull is at station +2 or more. Low forceps has two categories: if rotation is less than 45%, or if rotation is more than 45%, which should be stated when describing the low forceps category.

In the ACOG definitions, outlet forceps has been separated from low forceps. An outlet forceps is described as being present when the head is visible on the perineum (without manually separating the labia) and rotation beyond the oblique does not take place.

CLASSIFICATION OF FORCEPS BY PELVIC STATION AND VERTEX POSITION

Proposed Definitions

It is proposed that forceps be defined not as mid, low mid, low, or outlet forceps, but by pelvic station and position of vertex (Table 12.1).

For the remainder of this text, the use of the terms midforceps, low midforceps, or low forceps will be avoided. The reasoning for the new classification will be described in the next several paragraphs.

Implication of Station and Vertex Position in Forceps Classification

Station +3 and +4 are generally stations from which vaginal birth is expected. Vertex position, molding of the vertex, as well as maternal, fetal, and pelvic size influence the physician's expectations. At these lower positions cesarean delivery may not be easily accomplished as the lower uterine segment will be quite thin and fragile, and the low position of the vertex within the pelvis will necessitate force to return it to the abdomen. Many clinicians have spent a great deal of time resuturing the lower uterine segment, which literally falls apart after a long labor, followed by a difficult abdominal extraction of the fetus from a low pelvic station, performed in order to avoid use of the low midforceps.

The new forceps descriptive terminology by vertex, station, and position, has several advantages. All reviewers will know what the operator means when the forceps are described as station *(S)+2, vertex LOA.* This statement describes not only pelvic position but also implies a degree of

TABLE 12.1 Proposed Forceps Classification

Station	Vertex Position
0	OA, LOA, ROA, LOT, ROT, LOP, ROP, OP
+1	OA, LOA, ROA, LOT, ROT, LOP, ROP, OP
+2	OA, LOA, ROA, LOT, ROT, LOP, ROP, OP
+3	OA, LOA, ROA, LOT, ROT, LOP, ROP, OP
+4	OA, LOA, ROA, LOT, ROT, LOP, ROP, OP
+5	OA, LOA, ROA, LOT, ROT, LOP, ROP, OP

Abbreviations: O, occiput; A, anterior; L, left; R, right; T, transverse; P, posterior.

difficulty if forceps are used. Compare this statement to S+4 vertex LOA, and the conclusions are obvious. The clinician expects less difficulty or need for traction to be applied at a lower pelvic station. In classic terminology, both forceps would be considered midforceps, but only the classification by station describes the degree of traction and the degree of difficulty that may be present. Furthermore, investigators reviewing charts and attempting to determine at what pelvic station forceps application may increase morbidity for mother or fetus, could compare pelvic stations and vertex positions. In most studies, including the Cleveland forceps study, this information is not easily obtained. In many chart notes, forceps are often categorized low or mid, yet pelvic station may not be mentioned.

GUIDELINES FOR FORCEPS USE

Station

If, after vaginal examination, it is the clinician's judgment that the forceps birth will be difficult, even when it is known that the procedure can be accomplished, do not proceed. For obvious reasons, difficult forceps should be avoided unless, in the physician's judgment, cesarean birth or further time cannot be allowed. Forceps at station 0 and +1 are considered difficult and are generally replaced by allowing for more time in labor, if acceptable, or by cesarean if more time for labor is not acceptable. *Station +2* is generally a transition point in judgment for forceps use. Data relating to morbidity at different midpelvic stations is not available. Some obstetricians will deliver at this station; others feel that lack of experience does not allow a choice. Vertex position obviously should influence the decision. Forceps rotations from vertex positions other than the anterior position infer more difficulty.

Forceps use at stations +4 or +5 should be obvious. At those stations it is difficult to conceive of not delivering a vertex vaginally from any vertex position, including transverse and posterior. Station +4 should not be elective forceps use but warranted because of patient progress or fetal needs. Station +5 forceps use may be for various reasons, but it is primarily for maternal assistance.

Flexion

Flexion of the vertex facilitates passage of a smaller diameter of the vertex and foreshadows an easier birth. Without good flexion expect more difficulty. To flex the vertex with forceps is a procedure which must be taught in the delivery room. The position of the anterior and posterior fontanels, and whether the forceps blades at their heel or shanks are about two fingerbreadths below the posterior fontanel, needs to be noted during forceps application. If the shanks of the forceps are not in this position, the clinician may flex the vertex by opening, reapplying, and depressing the forceps blades so that the vertex will be flexed and come through the pelvis with a smaller diameter; therefore requiring less traction.

Asynclitism

Asynclitism, or lateral vertex flexion, is associated with a more difficult forceps application and more difficult delivery. Lateral flexion is corrected after the forceps application has begun. In contrast to actively flexing the head and changing forceps position in a deflexed head, asynclitism is corrected as the forceps blades are applied while attempting to lock the blades. At this point the clinician will find that one blade is higher on the vertex than its counterpart. Locking of the blades cannot take place until the forceps blades are manipulated to have equal length while correcting the lateral flexion of the vertex. If fenestrated forceps are being used, more of the fenestration (window) will be apparent on the side that must be deflexed. As the forceps blade is elevated and locked, the asynclitism is usually corrected. Asynclitism suggests more difficulty in forceps application and traction.

The Sacrum

If, during the vaginal examination, the hollow of the sacrum is easily felt behind the vertex, the vertex is either quite small or at much higher station than the operator anticipated. Discovering that there is room behind the vertex (in front of the sacrum) also implies that with further descent there should be more room in the pelvis for the vertex.

Vertex Position

The position of the vertex must be known. Without knowledge of at least the sagittal suture position, safe forceps application cannot be performed. The presence of the fontanels most easily indicates fetal position. When in doubt, search for an ear higher along the side of the vertex. The resistance of the back of the ear may help define the direction of the occiput. If the maternal abdomen has been examined earlier in labor, useful information will have been obtained. The back may have been palpated and also visualized as the straight side. The back and occiput should be on the same side. The information obtained from these earlier examinations may confirm an uncertain vaginal examination.

Vertex Molding

The long molded head found following a labor with a protracted active phase or a prolonged second stage should suggest that the vertex is at a higher pelvic station than it feels by palpation. A greater degree of difficulty with forceps use may be expected. Patients need to be evaluated in the context of the total labor picture, not just isolated pieces of information such as pelvic station or cervical dilatation.

Cervical Dilatation

The cervix must be fully dilated prior to applying forceps. In some cases the cervix will not disappear before vertex rotation takes place. The presence of a cervical rim or any palpable cervix along the side of the vertex suggests a more difficult procedure. Forceps use in these situations should be uncommon.

Fetal Size

The size of the fetus should be estimated by manual examination or by ultrasonography. Fetal size in general terms (large, average, or small) should have been estimated earlier in labor when the chart note was first written and the patient's labor was evaluated.

Pelvic Size

As stated earlier in this text, clinical estimation of pelvic size has been scorned by many clinicians and urged by others. At the first prenatal encounter with the patient, a pelvic estimate in general terms should be made. While the limitations of these measurements are understood, some general estimate is useful. In the delivery room, prior to forceps application, again attempt to review the patient's size and her clinical pelvimetry in association with the position of the vertex. These parameters are more meaningful if they are performed long before the patient's labor becomes complicated.

CLINICAL INDICATIONS FOR FORCEPS USE

In the previous section on guidelines for forceps use, some general assumptions were presented regarding information that should be known prior to the use of forceps. In this section on clinical indications for forceps, appropriate situations are presented when clinical choices and judgment, based on findings, come into play.

Fetal Distress

Fetal distress is an acceptable indication for forceps intervention. If, in the operator's judgment, fetal distress is present and some intervention should take place, forceps choice is acceptable. The clinical principles mentioned earlier apply. The sum of an equation, which balances fetal distress and potential trauma, needs to include an estimation of how serious the fetal distress may be, how rapidly the baby should be extracted (either by cesarean or forceps), and how difficult the forceps procedure is expected to be.

EXAMPLE OF POSSIBLE UMBILICAL CORD COMPRESSION

Following a normal labor a primigravid patient was 35 minutes into the second stage, fully dilated, with membranes ruptured, and at S+3 and vertex OA. Severe variable decelerations followed each contraction. The fetus was average in size. Clinical pelvimetry was felt to be normal. A fetal scalp blood sample revealed a mild respiratory acidosis with pH 7.21. Despite these findings, heart rate beat-to-beat variability appeared to be diminishing and the operator was concerned.

Comments

Although the situation was not yet critical, it was worrisome. Choices included waiting and repeating the scalp blood test, performing a cesarean, the use of midforceps, or vacuum extraction. The operator, believing the delivery to be relatively easy, chose to use Simpson forceps along with local anesthesia over a midline episiotomy. This clinical judgment is acceptable. The use of the vacuum or repetition of the scalp blood test would have been acceptable alternatives. There was no reason for a cesarean. According to the proposed terminology, this was an S+3 vertex OA forceps.

In some hospitals cesareans may be accomplished within 5 minutes from the time the crisis is detected. This level of support allows the clinician greater flexibility in treatment of choice. A forceps at station 0 may easily be replaced by a cesarean in the operator's judgment. In contrast, if 15 minutes or longer is required to effect delivery, the clinician's judgment of fetal risk may warrant vaginal forceps birth at all pelvic stations.

In describing acute situations such as fetal distress associated with abruption of the placenta or umbilical cord prolapse in the second stage of labor, once again evaluation of the reasons for the problem precedes clinical judgment and management. Although in this case forceps use is being discussed, in another instance the etiology of acute fetal distress may alter the clinician's consideration. A prolapsed umbilical cord may be treated first by vertex displacement, which may allow the operator more time to make a decision regarding a birth route choice. A placental separation is a very different problem.

Dystocia and Labor Abnormalities

In the presence of labor abnormalities, when time in seconds or minutes is not as critical, clinical judgment may be somewhat different. In labor abnormality situations, awaiting descent to lower stations and allowing more time in labor often will answer the problem and avoid the more difficult forceps. The difficult labor, followed by a forceps applied at stations +2 or +3, may foreshadow much more fetal risk than allowing an additional period of time to await further vertex descent. An arrest of descent at station +2 or +3 implies no similar urgency; this is in contrast to fetal distress, a situation in which length of time until delivery may be critical.

Arrest of Descent

The second stage of labor eventually must end, but, 1- or 2-hour time limits are arbitrary end points. Rather, the question should be whether progress is continuing or has descent arrested. If progress is continuing and time is not a problem (fetal distress is not present), the answer is easily reached: wait longer! If the patient needs more pain relief, use it.

Elective Forceps

Elective forceps is not an acceptable term. The use of forceps at any station is associated with some maternal and fetal risk. The term "elective" implies no presenting urgency for birth from maternal or fetal indications. If a mother is exhausted and the vertex is at station +4 or station +5, that is not an elective forceps use. Exhaustion needs treatment and forceps use or regional anesthesia are appropriate treatment choices.

In contrast, if epidural anesthesia has been given and rotation and descent appear to have ceased, then oxytocin, or allowing the epidural block to wear off, are more acceptable choices prior to forceps application.

Teaching Forceps

Teaching forceps is unacceptable; appropriate judgment should be taught. Forceps should not be applied electively in order to teach a resident. In those instances poor judgment is being taught.

The less frequent use of forceps in obstetrics suggests that experience in the use of forceps should be more focused in the later years of resident education. Forceps use above station +5 should be performed by residents in their senior years.

The number of forceps experiences which are needed by the resident in order to become comfortable and skilled in their use is a concern. The appropriate analogy is that the gynecology resident may perform 10, 15, or 25 vaginal hysterectomies before being considered adequately educated. Forceps experience depends on particular clinical conditions. Because forceps are less commonly used, their use must be taught well when it occurs. They should not be performed without the presence of an experienced clinician. All too often resident education is passed on from one resident to the next. Forceps use in many environments is too infrequent an occurrence to accept this learning method. Perhaps the learning of forceps should be treated with the same concern as the learning of difficult surgery. Certainly the implications in forceps use warrants this consideration.

The Low-Birth-Weight Fetus

The small fetus, categorized as the low-birth-weight (<2500 g) or very low-birth-weight (<1500 g) fetus, has been involved in the forceps debate for many years. Initially the debate involved the use of forceps in babies weighing 4 or 5 lb. It was never established whether, at those low birth weights, placing the fetal vertex in a "cage" to protect it from vaginal pressure or from too rapid expansion of the skull at birth produced improved results. Today, the data indicating forceps use for the very low-birth-weight fetus of less than 1500 g is even more limited. Forceps should be applied only if delivery needs to be effected because of clinical circumstances. Forceps are not a routine part of the care for the low-birth-weight fetus.

Even more controversial in this very low-birth-weight group is the suggestion by some clinicians that cesarean birth should be performed to improve fetal outcome and to prevent trauma or intracerebral fetal hemorrhage. At this time, there is no acceptable data documenting improved fetal outcome resulting from the cesarean birth route in the very low-birth-weight group. Birth of this more fragile fetus requires attention, the presence of an experienced clinician, and a controlled delivery, and that is the best clinical advice that can be offered until controlled studies are performed which test the hypothesis that change in birth route will improve outcome for the very low-birth-weight fetus.

The attempt to apply forceps to a low-birth-weight fetus is more easily decided upon than performed. When trying to apply forceps during a rapidly progressing labor, fetal position is often confusing. In the low-birth-weight fetus, because of the large fontanels and the soft skull, uncertainty of fetal position may lead to an attempt to apply forceps either too soon or too late. If applied too soon, there is a temptation to deliver the fetus from a higher station, and that is unacceptable. If applied too late, the head is born before the clinician is prepared. The important principle in birth technique for the low-birth-weight fetus is to control the rapidity of the birth of the head. This is effected by the presence of adequate perineal room provided by an episiotomy. The vertex should be born gradually, not abruptly. The clinician's hands should remain on the fetal vertex throughout the birth, and they should guide and control the descent and extension of the crowning vertex. It is not only vaginal muscle pressure on the fetal vertex that is a concern, but also too rapid expansion of the bones of the skull. If the head is born too rapidly, intracranial hemorrhage, such as dural sinus lacerations, may occur. Intracerebral bleeding in the low-birth-weight fetus appears to be more related to fetal maturity than to birth route choice.

TECHNICAL CONSIDERATIONS IN FORCEPS USE

Techniques taught in procedures such as forceps delivery or breech births are best taught in the delivery room. In the discussions on forceps, a philosophy and guideline for judgment has been presented. However, some statements may be made about the technical use of the forceps.

Types of Forceps

Since the use of forceps in most hospitals has been replaced with other methodologies, such as a tincture of time, the cesarean, or the vacuum extractor, technical skills are best acquired with simplified and standardized approaches to forceps use which may be repeated more frequently. If a Barton's or Kielland's forceps are rarely used, it is unlikely that adequate skill and confidence with these instruments will be retained. It is suggested that forceps use be limited to a few frequently used types.

A Simpson-type forceps with separated shanks should be appropriate for almost all births of the term size fetus during labor. For the smaller fetus, or the nonmolded fetal vertex, forceps with overlapping shanks will serve the rounder or smaller vertex. Rotations may be performed with these same forceps. If, in the clinician's judgment, the vertex position is too difficult to consider use of a Simpson-type forceps, it may perhaps be best not to use any forceps.

EXAMPLE OF BARTON FORCEPS OR NO FORCEPS

At term a normal-sized fetus presented with the cervix fully dilated, vertex LOT, station +2, and with a posterior parietal asynclitism. The Barton's forceps (with the anterior hinged blade) would have been an ideal instrument for delivery in this presentation.

Comment

Today, few clinicians can apply, rotate, and use traction with Barton's forceps. Because Barton's forceps are used infrequently, it may be best not to teach their use. Perhaps a vacuum extraction would be appropriate. Perhaps more time is needed. Appropriate forceps choice may be accomplished with a classical Simpson-type forceps, or if immediate delivery is warranted, a cesarean may be less traumatic than forceps. This is a judgment of the clinician's and, in part, depends on previous thinking.

Forceps Traction

Axis traction instruments are not recommended. If downward pressure on the forceps shanks and outward traction from the handle (known as the Pajot-Saxtorph maneuver) (Figure 12.1) does not allow descent of the vertex under the symphysis, perhaps too much force may be needed and the procedure should be reconsidered.The use of an axis traction instru-

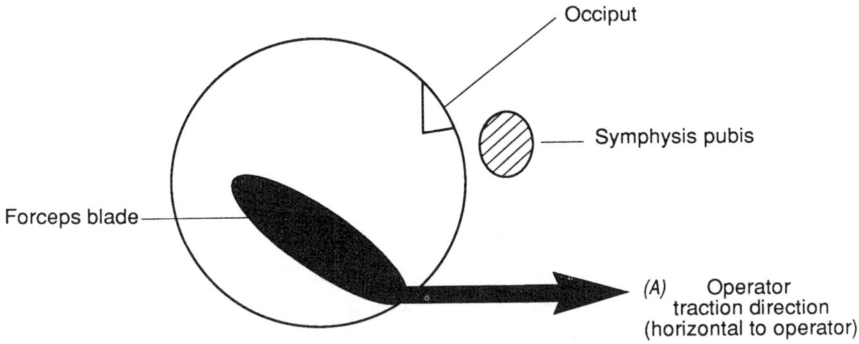

If traction is pulled towards the operator (A), the effective force (B) drives the occiput into the symphysis pubis. This is unacceptable.

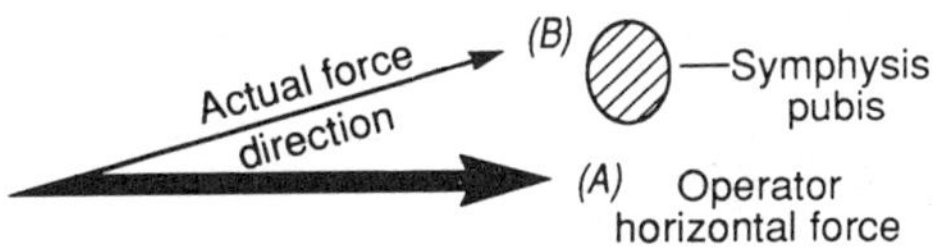

A way must be found to direct the vertex under the pubic symphysis. This is found by adding a second force (C) perpendicular to the floor that now changes the direction of the vertex (B).

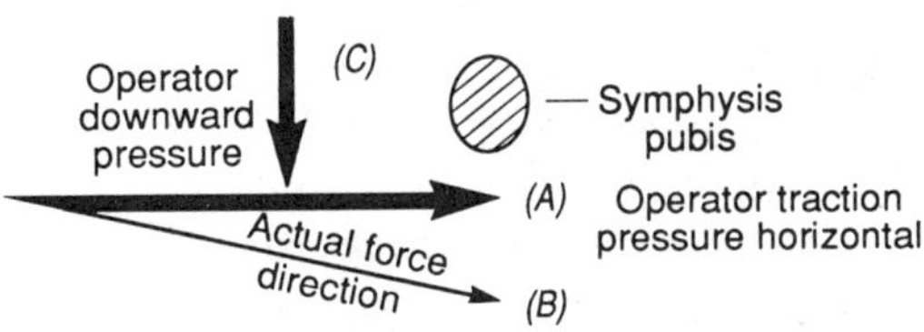

FIGURE 12.1

ment allows a great deal of force to be used without the operator sensing it during the traction.

Pelvic Curve and the Direction of Forceps Traction

To use traction, an understanding of the sacral pelvic curve with flexing of the occiput under the symphysis pubis is needed prior to extension of the vertex over the perineum. It is a common error for the operator to sit at the foot of the delivery table and, after the forceps application, apply horizontal traction towards the operator (Figure 12.1A and B). This is obviously incorrect. The downward *pressure on the forceps shanks* (Figure 12.1C) modulated with *the horizontal traction toward the operator* allows vertex descent toward the floor, under the pubic symphysis and the force vector or correct direction of the applied forces is achieved.

The ability to balance these two operator-applied forces allows a controlled vertex birth. At higher stations the operator must first use greater downward pressure on the forceps shanks. If during traction, particularly during forceps at stations +2 or +3, appropriate direction of the vertex under the symphysis pubis is not accomplished, greater force is required and greater pressure of the pubic symphysis on the skull occurs. Note again that these techniques are best taught in the delivery room when the delivery forces can be felt by the operator. Even the sitting position of the clinician on a stool at the foot of the delivery table is more easily understood when described in the delivery room. At that time the operator will understand why sitting on a low stool allows more efficient forceps traction at stations of the pelvis above +4 and +5.

Trial and Failed Forceps

These two terms represent a final attitude in a philosophy about forceps. If forceps are applied and it is discovered unexpectedly that they cannot be correctly applied, or after application in the delivery of the vertex in the operator's judgment acceptable traction is exceeded, it is wise to stop. That is a trial of forceps, or a failed forceps. To the less experienced obstetrician, how hard to pull with forceps and what is an acceptable application must be learned under the supervision of an experienced clinician. After several forceps applications, norms for acceptable traction are learned.

A procedure approached as "trial forceps" suggests uncertainty and anticipation of difficulty before starting. Reevaluate the situation. It does not take a great deal of humility to decide that more time in labor, oxytocin use, anesthesia, or a cesarean may be appropriate. A trial of forceps should be a very uncommon approach to patient care.

THE VACUUM EXTRACTOR

The nonrigid soft vacuum extraction instrument is in use in many areas of the world. Vacuum extraction of a fetus must be considered another mechanical traction instrument. It is useful, but it is not harmless. In general, indications for its use are similar to those of forceps. It is interesting to note that some reports document the use of the vacuum at higher stations and, on occasion, through an incompletely dilated cervix.[2]

Broekhuizen et al[2] noted vacuum extractions were being performed at higher stations—59.8% at station +1 or higher—compared with only 9% of forceps being used at similar stations. There appeared to be less maternal trauma although fetal skull fracture rates were similar when compared with forceps use at similar stations. The infants had a higher incidence of shoulder dystocia in the vacuum group. The major point to be made about the vacuum extractor is that while it is an acceptable technique to use, if indications for its use are expanded into areas already relinquished by forceps use, new data on morbidity will have to be collected. A conservative and less interventionist approach is suggested for the vacuum extractor, as with forceps.

SUMMARY

1. Forceps and the vacuum extractor are acceptable parts of obstetrical treatment.
2. Classification of forceps by station and position of the vertex should replace terminology for midforceps, low midforceps, low forceps, and outlet forceps.
3. Classification of forceps by five stations of the pelvis allows for comparison among forceps of comparable difficulty.
4. Forceps performed at stations 0 and +1 should be uncommon. The usually accepted transition point for forceps use appears to be pelvic station +2. It should be within the skills of the clinician to make a judgment choice for vaginal birth at stations +3, +4, and +5.
5. Forceps intervention should only be a final method for birth following appropriate labor trial or in the presence of fetal distress.
6. Forceps or cesarean birth are categories for terminating labor to be considered after other treatment modalities, such as time, ambulation, analgesia, oxytocin, and membrane rupture, have all been considered.
7. The introduction of the vacuum extractor should not be a license to perform more difficult mechanical deliveries.

REFERENCES

1. Committee in Obstetrics: Maternal and Fetal Medicine. Obstetric Forceps Committee Opinion Paper No. 59, American College of Obstetricians and Gynecologists, February, 1988.
2. Broekhuizen F, Washington J, Johnson F, Hamilton P: Vacuum extraction versus forceps delivery: indications and complications, 1979–1984. Obstet Gynecol 1987;69: 338–342.

Chapter 13

Breech Presentation

The Controversy

OVERVIEW

Perhaps even more controversial than forceps use, the problem of birth route choice for the breech presentation is clouded by emotions, including physician and patient anxieties, and confusion of outcome benefit as recorded in the literature. In 1981 in the United States more than 60% of all fetuses in breech position were delivered by cesarean.[1] The increasing trend toward cesarean birth for the breech presentation has continued well beyond the time of the 1981 National Institutes of Health report.[1] It is apparent at most institutions that if the mother can be taken to the operating room before vaginal birth occurs, the cesarean will be the birth route. There is also a movement by some hospital risk-management personnel to urge the use of the cesarean birth route to avoid any potential litigious consequences which may surround a breech fetus born vaginally. As in the cases of midforceps or fetal distress, in a breech birth, if morbidity develops during infancy or later in life, a search for etiology often returns to the birth process, even when data may suggest the birth process was not the problem.

The goal in this chapter is to demonstrate that, with respect to the breech presentation in labor, there is room for choice. It is important to understand why this controversy exists and why birth route choice is acceptable. To this end, the confounding variables in breech presentations which may make breech presentation an at-risk situation will be explored first. A breech presentation may also be associated with non-birth-route-incurred risks for neurological morbidity.

Data relating to the breech birth controversy will be discussed first, followed by a discussion of studies in the problematic area of vaginal versus cesarean birth route. A more complete discussion of when and how to deliver a breech fetus will be presented in Chapter 14.

OBJECTIVES

At the conclusion of this chapter, the clinician should:

1. Be aware of the literature describing birth route decisions for the breech presentation
2. Know the variables which will always confuse outcome in all breech presentations
3. Be able to individualize patient care in reaching a birth route choice in the frank breech position

CONFOUNDING VARIABLES IN THE BREECH PRESENTATION WHICH LEAD TO INCREASED INFANT MORBIDITY AND MORTALITY

Certain risks cannot be altered by changing the birth route. The question that should be considered by the clinician prior to making a birth route decision is: Why is this fetus in breech presentation? At times the breech presentation may represent an already present fetal neurologic problem which has altered fetal movement patterns or body shape.

Congenital Anomalies and Abnormalities

Major anomalies of the fetus are severalfold higher in breech presentations.[2] Examples are Potters syndrome with its abnormal fetal shape and absent kidneys, or congenital hydrocephalus with its enlarged fetal head. These examples are two among many conditions which have a higher than anticipated risk for breech presentation. Prior to reaching a clinical decision for birth route, ultrasonography is necessary for fetal evaluation. For example, in a fetus without kidneys, it would not be prudent to deliver that breech position fetus by cesarean if vaginal birth were possible without incurring harm to the mother.

In contrast to gross congenital anomalies, it is also documented that the normal-appearing fetus in breech presentation has a higher than expected incidence of genetically acquired mental and biochemical abnormalities.[3] These gene abnormalities cannot be seen with ultrasonography, but add to the already higher morbidity for the fetus in breech presentation.

Fetal Activity and Neurologic Function

More subtle and even more difficult to document is the thesis that fetal movement may be different in the breech presentation. In this speculation the vertex position may be assumed because of an already present neurologic abnormality which makes the breech presentation fetus move differently from the vertex-presenting fetus. This infers that some developmental or traumatic event has already taken place in the central nervous system.

Prematurity

As the fetus approaches term, the incidence of breech presentation decreases. In the low-birth-weight population, a higher incidence of the breech presentation is present, and infant outcome is intertwined with the risks of gestational immaturity. This is described more extensively in the following section on Debate in the Literature.

Other Confounding Variables

In association with low birth weight, we also find *premature rupture of the membranes* and *in utero infection* at higher incidence in the breech presentation. These obstetrical problems lead to higher morbidity and mortality irrespective of fetal position or birth route choice.

Adding to the confusion, in many breech studies, which usually are reviews of hospital's activities, *the stillbirth fetus* in breech presentation is always delivered vaginally. The live fetus in breech presentation is delivered by cesarean, again biasing some of the study numbers.

Risk Variables Intrinsic to the Breech Presentation During Labor

Fetal size, as in the large fetus, is a concern in all gestations but even more worrisome in the breech presentation. Concern for difficulty in extracting the fetal shoulders or fetal head lead most clinicians to consider cesarean birth.

Similarly in the small fetus, a disproportionately large head compared with abdomen and shoulder size increases the concern for fetal head entrapment. A smaller presenting part that does not fill the pelvis well increases the risk for prolapse of the umbilical cord. In comparison with the earlier confounding variables, these risks are associated primarily with vaginal birth. In the breech presentation some risks, such as prolapsed umbilical cord, may occur quite early in labor onset, occurring with spontaneous membrane rupture even before the patient reaches the hospital.

DEBATE IN THE LITERATURE

Hall et al[4] reviewed the breech presentation and perinatal mortality over a 10-year period beginning in 1950. The authors presented data during a time when physicians' attitudes were evolving toward more frequent use of cesareans for many obstetrical problems. These authors noted the high incidence of low-birth-weight fetuses in the breech category. Twenty-four percent to 30% of all breech presentations weighed between 1000 g and 2500 g. The authors also confirmed that in the second 5 years of their report there was a 50% increase in breech cesarean birthrate, reaching a high of 15.1% of births by cesarean for the breech fetus. The high perinatal loss in the study associated with breech presentation was in part accounted for by low birth weight. In their conclusions, the authors stated that an increased risk for breech birth exists with vaginal birth, and urged the presence of an experienced physician when breech labor occurs.

In commenting on the paper by Hall et al,[4] which was presented at a meeting of the American Association of Obstetricians and Gynecologists in 1964, Robert A. Cosgrove, MD, noted his concern about the increasing use of cesareans, as breech presentations, resulted in cesarean sections 20% of the time at the Margaret Hayes Maternity Hospital where he was the director. These two commentaries documented the changing attitudes toward breech birth and the mixed judgment philosophies in this difficult obstetrical clinical decision.

Berendes et al,[5] using sophisticated statistical approaches to the problem, attempted to determine the priority of importance of risk factors for both mortality and morbidity from the large number of breech births in the Collaborative Study of Cerebral Palsy. They found, among other risks, the strong influence of both congenital anomalies and birth weight on breech outcomes.

By the mid-1970s most fetuses in breech presentation were being delivered by cesarean. In a report by DeCrespigny and Pepperell,[6] justification for the increased use of cesareans for the mature breech fetus (>2500 g) was questioned. The authors noted no increase in survival in the breech population when delivered by cesarean. Duenholter et al,[7] in a controlled study during the same time period, suggested that the abdominal route was safer for the low-birth-weight fetus (between 1000 and 2500 g). Discussing term infants, Mann and Gallant[8] reviewed 457 breech births and failed to find a significant decrease in mortality or morbidity in the breech fetus born by the cesarean birth route when compared to the vaginal route.

Graves[9] presented data derived from the analysis of breech births between the years 1957 and 1976 in a partnership private practice. In that restricted clinical environment, the fetus below 2500 g appeared to benefit from a cesarean birth. Graves noted equivocal findings for the over 2500-g fetus. He also discussed the impact of the "current torts situation" on physician decision making. Today increased legal risk is an accepted fact of the practicing obstetrician. Thus in the breech presentation, clinical decisions will be influenced not only by what is best for the fetus and mother, but also by which choice poses less risk for the clinician.

In an almost unique prospective study which took place between 1975 and 1979, Collea et al[10] set stringent management guidelines, including the use of x-ray pelvimetry, and accomplished a randomized trial of vaginal and cesarean birth routes for the frank breech presentation. In their conclusions the authors supported vaginal delivery for term frank breech births, and noted that even when the breech presentation in labor was randomized into the cesarean birth route, they could not get all patients to the operating room in time to do the cesarean.

The unresolved debate has continued into the 1980s. Petitti and Golditch[11] described a large private practice group health plan and reported on all birth weights over 1000 g. No demonstrable mortality differences with respect to birth route choice were found. In a study by Bodmer et al,[12] the increased cesarean rate did not reduce severe respiratory depression at birth in breech presentation, which is always higher in the breech than in the cephalic presentation. Birth trauma and encephalopathy, when compared with earlier studies, remained the same. The authors cautioned that head entrapment in the under 1000-g population was responsible for 7 deaths of 55 live-born infants, and cesarean was performed least frequently in that population.

DATA FROM THE CLEVELAND STUDY

Influenced in part by rising cesarean births in general, and by the preponderance of cesareans for the breech presentation, a retrospective review of breech birth outcomes at Cleveland Metropolitan General Hospital during the 1970s was undertaken to review neurologic morbidity.[13] The study took place in an environment where birth route choice still existed for the fetus in frank breech presentation. Consultation between patient and physician involved trying to reach a decision as to birth route choice. Despite the flexibility for birth route choice in association with this process, more than 60% of breech presentations were delivered by cesarean. The clinical staff was no different in their attitudes toward the breech than attitudes present in most hospitals.

In the Cleveland retrospective review for neonatal morbidity and mortality, when breech presentations within comparable weight groups were compared, neonatal neurologic morbidity was not decreased by choice for cesarean.[13] When assessing the data within comparable weight groups, it was of interest to note that most breech presentations in labor were born vaginally in the 500- to 750-g category. Above 750 g, the cesarean became the birth route of choice. This implies a new confounding variable which must be considered in the evaluation of all nonrandomized breech studies.

It is apparent that if the physician thinks the fetus is viable, he or she is most likely to treat the fetus differently and this affects outcome. In the Cleveland study, fewer cesareans were performed for the very lowest birth weights when the baby was felt to be nonviable. Thus, if one reviewed overall neonatal risk rather than comparing outcome within small birth categories, the higher incidence of vaginal birth route for low-birth-weight fetuses would inevitably bias the review against the vaginal birth route.

It must also be noted that the lack of accurate gestational age or weight prediction methods confounded many study outcomes. In all nonrandomized studies a nonmeasurable variable, important in birth route selection, was the physician's expectation of fetal viability, adding to the confusion of outcomes in breech presentations. If the physician expected that the breech was of sufficient size to survive, it was born by surgery; if expected to be previable it was born vaginally. Yet inability to predict viability allowed the very low-birth-weight populations to be treated with different expectations in the vaginal group.

Because in the first Cleveland breech study neurologic morbidity was not easily diagnosed before the infants left the nursery, a prospective study was performed to determine infant neurologic outcomes at age 2-years. The vaginally born frank breech presentation was matched by birth weight, with a vaginally born vertex, a cesarean born vertex, and a cesarean born breech of similar birth weights.[14] In this quadruple match, major fetal congenital anomalies and in utero fetal deaths prior to arriving at the hospital were excluded. The results confirmed that the morbidity for the frank breech presentation born vaginally was no different than that for the breech born by cesarean of comparable birth weight.

Following both studies, it was clear that morbidity may be influenced by many factors, but the most important factor was the maturity of the fetus.[13,14] While entrapment of the head and prolapse of the umbilical cord did occur, the frequencies of these events were so low and apparently so well recognized (the prolapsed umbilical cord) that these often spoken of fears were not major factors in infant morbidity or mortality. This understanding has led to a philosophy, as expressed in the Chapter 14, that birth route choice is acceptable as a treatment option for the fetus in labor as a frank breech presentation. In addition, if the fact that no morbidity differences were apparent at any birth weight, the proposition that cesarean birth for the very low-birth-weight fetus remains undocumented. This also removes the need to guess expected fetal birth weight before deciding birth route for the low-birth-weight fetus. That is, should a cesarean be performed for the less than 2500-g fetus or the less than 1000-g fetus as reported in some studies?

Today the birth route choice controversy continues. More frequently authors consider, on the basis of their findings, vaginal delivery for the frank breech presentation weighing more than 2500 g. Other birth weight windows for cesarean birth often exclude the lowest birth weights on the basis of viability and the over 4000-g fetus on the basis of size.

Based on data obtained from the Cleveland programs birth route choice for the frank breech presentation will be presented as an acceptable option for the clinician to offer the patient. This option exists at all birth weights below 4000 g. The Cleveland studies did not have sufficient data to comment on birth weights above 4000 g.

SUMMARY

1. Today, the majority of frank breech presentations are delivered by cesarean.
2. The literature documents conflicting opinions based on data for breech births at all birth weights.
3. Confounding variables, important in understanding the literature and in reaching a clinical birth route choice in frank breech presentations, include congenital anomalies, prematurity, and preexisting fetal brain damage.
4. At the lowest birth weights, when viability is not expected, most breech births are born vaginally.
5. Despite the increased cesarean birthrate, continuing reduction in infant morbidity is not demonstrated.
6. It is proposed that, at all birth weights, there is an acceptable argument for birth either vaginally or abdominally, and the choices should be reviewed with the patient prior to reaching a decision.

REFERENCES

1. Cesarean Childbirth, publication 82-2067. Bethesda, MD, National Institutes of Health, October 1981, pp 375–386.
2. Brenner WE: Breech presentation. Clin Obstet Gynecol 1978;21:511–513.
3. Braun FH, Jones KL, Smith DW: Breech presentation as an indicator of fetal abnormality. J Pediatr 1975;86:419–421.
4. Hall JE, Kohl SK, O'Brien F, Ginsberg M: Breech presentation and perinatal mortality. Am J Obstet Gynecol 1965;91:665–683.

5. Berendes HW, Weiss W, Deutschberger J, Jackson E: Factors associated with breech delivery. Am J Public Health 1965;55:708–719.
6. DeCrespigny LJC, Pepperell RJ: Perinatal mortality and morbidity in breech presentation. Obstet Gynecol 1979;53:141–145.
7. Duenholter JH, Wells CE, Reich JS, Santos Ramos R, Jimenez J: A paired controlled study of vaginal and abdominal delivery of the low birth weight breech fetus. Obstet Gynecol 1979;54;310–313.
8. Mann LI, Gallant JM: Modern management of breech delivery. Am J Obstet Gynecol 1979;134:611–614.
9. Graves WK: Breech delivery in twenty years of practice. Am J Obstet Gynecol 1980;137:229–234.
10. Collea JV, Chein C, Quilligan EJ: The randomized management of term frank breech presentation: a study of 208 cases. Am J Obstet Gynecol 1980;137:235–244.
11. Petitti DB, Golditch IM: Mortality in relation to method of delivery in breech infants. Int J Gynecol Obstet 1984;22:189–193.
12. Bodmer B, Benjamin A, McClean FH, Usher PH: Has the use of cesarean section reduced the risks of delivery in the preterm breech presentation? Am J Obstet Gynecol 1986;154:244–250.
13. Rosen MG, Chik L: The effect of delivery route on outcome in breech presentation. Am J Obstet Gynecol 1984;148:909–914.
14. Rosen MG, Debanne S, Thompson K, Bilenker RM: Long term neurological morbidity in breech and vertex births. Am J Obstet Gynecol 1985;151:718–720.

Chapter 14

Breech Presentation

Delivery

OVERVIEW

It should be apparent from the review in Chapter 13 that clinically it is still appropriate to consider vaginal delivery for the frank breech presentation. Yet the clinician should not underestimate nor minimize the potential medical and emotional risks to both patient and physician when considering the vaginal birth route. In the already presented information it was documented that routine use of the cesarean birth route did not avoid all the risks inherent in the frank breech presentation. Birth weight and maturity appeared to be far more important than birth route in infant neurologic outcome[1,2] and, despite the increased use of the cesarean, decrease in breech presentation morbidity was not apparent.[3] In this chapter patient evaluation prior to choosing the birth route, and patient management, prior to and during labor, will be presented.

OBJECTIVES

At the conclusion of this chapter, the clinician should be able to:

1. Understand the guidelines for external breech version prior to labor
2. Present options to the patient for management of the frank breech presentation
3. Provide management plans for the frank breech presentation prior to labor
4. Better understand some of the mechanics for frank breech birth

EVALUATION PRIOR TO LABOR

The Initial Visit

The initial visit is reemphasized as a general approach to all patients. Assess the patient physically and emotionally during the first visit, including a general appraisal of body size and shape. A patient 4 ft 10 in tall is of concern no matter what her fetal presentation is at term. A patient with an abnormal walking gait may have an asymmetrically shaped pelvis. Clinical measurement of the pelvis should be conducted. These patient care variables are not as objectively assessed during active labor and are best conducted during early pregnancy. Knowing that a fetus is in breech presentation may alter the clinician's objectivity if pelvimetry and clinical assessment are carried out for the first time.

Information in the antepartum records should describe the initial findings, and an estimate should have been made that a normal size fetus may traverse the pelvis. In a contrasting example, clinical findings describing a flat or forward sacrum during the patient's first visit will be of major importance during labor.

If, in the presence of a breech presentation at the time of labor, review of the initial visit suggests limited pelvic capacity, avoid the vaginal route. There should be no trial of labor in breech presentation in this case. Pelvic capacity is not tested until the fetal head is born. The key thought expressed here is that clinical estimates are assessed prior to the breech position risk. Obviously the patient will need to be reevaluated in the new situation, but in the presence of the breech, having the information already in place supports a more objective approach.

Patient Emotional State and Patient Involvement in the Decision

Consider the patient's emotional state and her wishes. Some couples come to the physician with outspoken desires for birth route choice and labor management, others depend on the physician to make the medical decision. There is great diversity. Some patients may be better able to work with physicians during labor and sustain clinical "crises." Others have more difficulty responding in a constructive way to a difficult labor decision.

EXAMPLE OF PATIENT REQUEST FOR EXTERNAL VERSION

The physician received a phone call from a multipara at 39 weeks of gestation. The caller asked to have an external breech version performed so that a vertex presentation could be obtained. The physician had not seen the patient previously. The patient wished to return to her midwife and deliver vaginally at home. The patient was not reassured by the physician's responses over the phone and she chose to go elsewhere.

Comment

If an external version is performed the clinician should take responsibility for the vaginal delivery or at least insist that the birth take place in a hospital environment. Often there is a continuum of risk for the breech presentation and preexisting problems incurred prior to labor may be present. The breech, even when turned to a vertex, may represent an already present risk for neurologic maturity. In addition, a return to the breech position following a successful version may occur. The fetus is at risk and should not be considered for a home delivery.

EXAMPLE OF PHYSICIAN BIASING PATIENT CHOICE

A multiparous patient at 39 weeks gestation was told of the frank breech presentation of the fetus and offered a choice of vaginal or abdominal birth. She obtained a second opinion from an obstetrician who stated that all breech presentations should be delivered by cesarean. She remained with the second obstetrician who delivered her fetus by cesarean.

Comment

It is evident that on consultation with a second physician, choice was not offered to the patient. It is also apparent that this patient did not wish to make a choice but desired that the obstetrician make the decision. In this example, the offering of a choice for birth route was not acceptable to the patient.

Patient Information

The ground rules for this higher risk situation should be clear. Medical information should be exchanged and discussed when the breech presentation is noted and the physician should have a chart note documenting the exchange. Should a breech presentation be found first at 30 weeks gestation or at a first early visit, the presentation should be reconfirmed at the next visit. As breech presentation incidence is highest earlier in gestation, it should be reconfirmed at a later visit. If the breech persists, it is time to discuss the facts about breech births and the available options. Although the breech may change to a vertex, the information needs to be discussed at a nonstressful time.

In contrast to the breech presentation found earlier in pregnancy which usually changes to a vertex presentation during the next several visits, the breech presentation near term should be discussed with the patient when first found. It may, but usually does not, convert to a vertex presentation at or near term.

Although clinical studies suggest that vaginal birth is appropriate, patient choice should be encouraged in this medical situation. If the patient has strong fears or rejects the vaginal route, it is suggested that the clinician should not pursue the issue. The emotional and medicolegal implications are too overwhelming for the physician to be arbitrary.

Antepartum Considerations

Leopold's maneuvers should be performed for all pregnancies at each patient visit after 24 weeks of gestation. If a breech presentation is suspected, ultrasonography should be performed to document the breech and the absence of major congenital anomalies. The breech presentation confirmed prior to labor allows for more discussion with the patient.

The Antepartum Preterm Breech

It is suggested that between 24 and 36 weeks, ultrasonography be ordered at the first detection of the breech presentation. As noted, the breech is more common in incidence early in pregnancy and usually converts to a vertex presentation spontaneously. There is no purpose in alarming the patient. When the breech persists at a second visit, discussions with the patient should begin and ultrasonography should be scheduled. Persistence of the breech presentation for two visits may indicate a reason for the position, rather than a chance occurrence.

The purpose of ultrasonography is to rule out fetal anatomic defects which may be incompatible with life or incompatible with vaginal birth. If a major congenital anomaly is found, or if sufficient time remains, amniocentesis or fetal umbilical cord sampling for the fetal karyotype may document syndromes incompatible with life. These findings would alter the birth route choice. Umbilical fetal blood sampling is available in some centers and may be considered if time for karyotyping of amniotic fluid is not available. These vascular studies can be analyzed within days. Fetal karyotype studies are not suggested for the breech presentation fetus in the absence of morphologic anomalies.

VERSION OF THE TERM BREECH

External Version

From 37 weeks to term, external version should be considered in an attempt to obtain a vertex presentation. More physicians are gaining experience with this technique. Most authors, when reporting on their experience, suggest turning the breech fetus between 36 and 37 weeks.[4] As term approaches, increase in fetal size, decrease in amniotic fluid, and lower pelvic position of the breech make version more difficult.

Version Site

External cephalic version should be performed in an environment where a response to unexpected fetal distress during the version may be undertaken rapidly. Umbilical cord problems may be aggravated by the version maneuvers, for example, if the cord is already around a limb or the neck. The use of ultrasonography may allow the clinician to anticipate umbilical cord problems during the procedure. For example, coils of umbilical cord around the neck or limbs may be seen. If bradycardia ensues, the reasons will be clear and the clinical response to discontinue the version will be rapid. Placental separation may occur secondary to the abdominal pressure exerted during the procedure although this is uncommon. If the patient is Rh-negative, it is possible that sensitization may take place. The use of Rhogam should be considered. Even if Rhogam has already been given at 28 weeks of gestation, additional blocking antibody may be needed if an unusual fetal hemorrhage occurred following the manipulation. There is no data in this area that suggests major fetal hemorrhagic risk.

Uterine Muscle Relaxants

Most version techniques use uterine muscle relaxants such as Ritodrine or Terbutaline. Some clinicians have used muscle and patient relaxants such as Valium. Sufficient amniotic fluid must be present. An external version cannot be performed in the presence of ruptured membranes.

Techniques

Techniques for version are best taught at the bedside, and they are described in standard texts. In general, in the external version one may attempt to turn the head of the fetus forward over its heels. If that does not work, the reverse direction is tried. Constant steady upward pressure is maintained with one hand on the breech elevating it out of the pelvis. At times the breech is so low in the pelvis that the version becomes difficult or impossible. A rotary motion in the direction of the turn is used on the head and back with the other hand. Try to spin the breech around as if following the circumference of a circle. The maternal abdomen should be well lubricated with powder or oil so that the hands move easily in the direction in which the clinician is attempting to turn the breech. This procedure may take 5 to 15 minutes. Try to continue ultrasonography at all times during the procedure in order to visualize progress and to follow the fetal heart rate. If unsuccessful in the version, discontinue the procedure. Not all breeches will be turned. Morrison et al[4] noted reasonable success with an overall lowering of the incidence of breech births at term.

Following the external version, continuous fetal monitoring for the next hour is recommended. Bradycardia of a transient nature often occurs during the version.

EXAMPLE OF THE NEED FOR RULING OUT FETAL DISTRESS

A version of breech to vertex took place without difficulty followed by normal postversion electronic heart rate monitoring. Later an uncomplicated delivery of the infant in vertex position took place. At 48 hours of age, the neonate convulsed. There was no evidence for an etiology for the convulsion.

Comment

The question persists as to whether neonatal convulsions reflected trauma incurred at the time of the version, or if the trauma was already present in the fetus in the breech presentation. Preexisting breech risk has been described in Chapter 13. It was reassuring to the clinician to be able to confirm that no fetal cardiac abnormalities were present during the version or afterwards.

DECISIONS DURING LABOR

Since it is almost impossible to prepare a patient for every medical possibility, and the breech may not be diagnosed until labor onset, discussion about the problems and alternatives of the breech birth take place in a much more difficult environment.

In the labor room, faced with the emotions of labor plus an unexpected clinical finding, it is more difficult to offer choices to the patient or family and have those choices acted upon in an objective manner. Nevertheless, to the greatest extent possible, family consultation is important. The guidelines for care do not change. Discuss and obtain the same kind of permission as would be obtained for any intervention during labor, and record in the patient's chart the fact that the discussion took place and the conclusions reached at that time.

EXAMPLE OF UNEXPECTED BREECH PRESENTATION DURING LABOR

A patient was in her fifth pregnancy with a benign past medical and obstetrical history. Labor began 3 hours before arrival at the hospital. A frank breech in LST position at S+1 and full dilatation was found. The estimated fetal size was 7 lb. The patient was beginning to push with each contraction. There was no evidence of fetal distress. She was told of the situation and immediately taken to the delivery room. Thirty-five minutes later she spontaneously vaginally delivered a normal infant over a midline episiotomy.

Comment

A decision had to be made rapidly in a high-tension situation. It was clear that the new findings in labor left little room for an objective patient choice. In this example, the obstetrician assumed responsibility for the medical decision based on the judgment that a normal rapid delivery was anticipated. Unfortunately, someone could argue years later that the 35 minutes of time which elapsed would have enabled the clinician to perform a cesarean. While this may be true, in the prospective management of the breech this could not have been anticipated. This is a time in which the clinician must assume full responsibility and make a decision based on his or her best medical judgment.

THE HOSPITAL ENVIRONMENT

The ability of a hospital to be able to rapidly perform a cesarean for fetal distress or for other unexpected maternal or fetal problems is important. If a management decision is made for a vaginal birth, all support systems for birth route should be in place. Supports include the availability of an operating room, anesthesia support, and the presence of a pediatrician. When these support persons are not available, choices become less flexible.

In some hospitals, at late hours, additional staff normally take calls from home. If possible, when the diagnosis is made, choose to bring staff to the hospital to be present throughout labor. As stated before in this text, if there is a choice between hospitals for delivery in the region, whenever possible, the higher-risk patient should be delivered in the higher-level patient care environment. In addition, prior to being booked for delivery at a hospital, the patient needs to know the different capabilities of the available hospitals.

X-RAY PELVIMETRY

X-ray pelvimetry has little predictive value. Having said that, if possible perform x-ray pelvimetry for the breech (not for the vertex). In the presence of a normal pelvis, proceed. The logic for a decision to desist from vaginal birth, based on x-ray pelvimetry, cannot be defended any better for the breech than for the vertex. However, noting the many medical and legal pitfalls of the breech birth, it is easier to state to all later questioners that the pelvimetry was normal rather than to defend its absence. If x-ray pelvimetry is not desired or unavailable, depend on the clinical evaluation.

COMPUTERIZED AVERAGE TOMOGRAPHY OF THE PELVIS

Computerized average tomography has been suggested as being useful, and more accurate than x-ray pelvimetry and it incurs a lower dose of radiation for both breech and vertex presentations.[5] Tomography may demonstrate a better correlation between fetal head size and pelvis, and the measurements may be more accurate. Data on the usefulness of this test, evaluated by controlled clinical studies is not available. In the end, however, it is usually not size that is the problem of the breech birth, it is the adaptation of the upper body and aftercoming head to the pelvis. Radiography will not likely foreshadow those events.

INTRAPARTUM CARE

At the start of labor, a flat film of the abdomen or ultrasonography should be used to demonstrate that the head is not hyperextended. If hyperextended early in labor, the head is more likely to stay in that position during the final phase of delivery. This larger diameter makes for a difficult and potentially traumatic birth. If the head is flexed at the start of the labor, it is less likely to change. In the presence of hyperextension of the fetal head, it is prudent to perform a cesarean. Even with a cesarean the clinician must be aware of birth mechanics as vertex hyperextension may also lead to a more difficult extraction from the uterus.

The Low-Birth-Weight Fetus

At all fetal birth weight estimates vaginal birth is an acceptable choice for the frank breech presentation (see Chapter 13). Extraction of a low-birth-weight breech from a cesarean incision is also potentially traumatic. Because choice is acceptable at all fetal weights, the problem of estimating size for the small fetus is less important than the question of previability.

Electronic Fetal Monitoring

Perhaps it is unnecessary to state, but for completeness, continuous electronic fetal monitoring is part of the breech surveillance process. The risk of umbilical cord compression, one of the two major risks to the breech in labor (the second is delivery of the aftercoming head), can be recognized and responded to. External monitoring is acceptable if the data is useful. If not, the electrode can be inserted into the fetal buttock.

Intravenous Fluids

Intravenous fluids and an open emergency line to the patient are not warranted in all low-risk labors. Choice by the patient is acceptable. However, intravenous lines should be used for the frank breech woman in labor to allow for response to emergencies, such as a need for rapid induction of anesthesia.

Pain Medications

Treat a breech birth with pain medication the same as with all other births. If pain medication is needed, analgesia or regional blocks may be used. As with all labor patients, minimal medication and spontaneous birth is preferred. Arguments have been written supporting the use of many forms of medication and regional blocks. No single special medication exists in this area.[6] Individualize patient care and choose the mode of pain relief that the changing circumstances warrant. If the fetus is of low birth weight, concern as to type of medication is more important. Many clinicians prefer to have the patient deliver the fetus spontaneously and without regional block anesthesia, but this is not a universal opinion. Regional blocks can be given which allow the patient to assist in the breech birth.

Oxytocin Use

With each additional complication that may occur, the prudent physician often refrains from vaginal birth and proceeds to cesarean. In the presence of breech birth, the use of oxytocin is not usually encouraged. Oxytocin may be used infrequently and only in the presence of poor contractions or poor progress. However, there is little evidence in any controlled studies supporting a mandated standard of care. In the presence of a normal size mother and fetus, oxytocin stimulation of labor after spontaneous membrane rupture or augmentation of labor is not contraindicated.

BREECH BIRTH MECHANICS

There is no single or best method for delivering the frank breech vaginally. Several general guidelines are suggested.

Anesthesia

In the case of the breech birth adequate support personnel should be present. An anesthesiologist or anesthetist should be present at the head of the table and able to administer rapid, complete anesthesia if it is needed. It is important for the patient to know that these events may take place. It is also important to convey to the anesthesiologist that there may be a need for a surgical level of anesthesia with complete muscular and uterine relaxation. Analgesia will not help if a manipulative delivery occurs and the cervix is clamped around the fetal head. All management considerations should be planned ahead with the patient and support staff.

Neonatal Care

Where possible, staff able to provide respiratory support for the neonate should be present. Although respiratory problems are not usual they should be anticipated. The breech presentation is a high-risk labor, and someone should be available to deliver care to the neonate.

Obstetrical Support

As in a cesarean, when possible, it is helpful to have a second clinician present. That person should palpate the fetal vertex at the start of the delivery and follow it abdominally as it descends into the pelvis and the birth takes place. This individual maintains gentle but continuing pressure on the fetal head in order to maintain flexion and to prevent extension of the aftercoming head as it descends into the pelvis from complicating the birth. As the birth occurs it may also be necessary to ask for more suprapubic pressure to deliver the head by flexing it into the pelvis if the maternal expulsion efforts are not effective. Knowing where the vertex is at the start and throughout the delivery can facilitate this procedure.

Patience

When the breech is near, the clinician should not help it along. Do not begin to extract or pull it down because it can be reached and progress is not as rapid as anticipated. Rapid deliveries lead to nuchal arms and extended heads. Listen to the monitor, encourage the mother, be patient, do not intervene.

Episiotomy

As the breech crowns, birth can be facilitated by an episiotomy. Perform a midline incision with the use of local anesthesia. If necessary, the episiotomy may be extended into the rectum and repaired as a fourth-degree laceration.

Fetal Body Support

As the breech is born, there is a general tendency to extract it. Instead support the breech and the abdomen as the birth progresses. The word "support" is emphasized rather than "to pull." At the same time the mother is encouraged to continue to deliver the fetus spontaneously. A spontaneous breech birth with controlled expression of the aftercoming head is always attempted before any intervention.

The Umbilical Cord

Many authors suggest that as the abdomen appears the operator should reach up for the umbilical cord and be sure it is pulsating. That is always reassuring; however, the electronic monitor should still be in place. Do not stop monitoring electronically on arrival to the delivery room.

By the time the umbilicus is reached, the cord will be easily available for palpation. It often is difficult for an anxious obstetrician to be certain if it is the cord pulsations which are felt during the delivery or the obstetrician's trembling fingers. However, when the umbilicus is reached, do not expect to delay. The birth should continue to move forward.

The Shoulders and Arms

While shoulders may be a problem in a vertex birth, they generally are not the major problem in the breech birth. If spontaneous birth appears slow, traction applied to the body may be needed; then deliver one or both arms if they are nuchal. There is no reason, in a progressing birth, to intervene unless progress has stopped. It is important to allow the aftercoming head to enter the pelvis slowly. If traction is needed, it should be used along with synchronous suprapubic pressure on the fetal head. Traction may be applied from the fetal ankles or thighs and presacral region. This is a matter of choice.

If the fetal arms are nuchal, attempt to sweep them down by applying pressure along the fetal humerus with an index finger. Attempt to deliver the anterior arm first. If that fails, then reach for the posterior arm. If neither arm is easily reached, attempt to rotate the trunk 180° in whichever direction appears easiest.

If only one arm is nuchal and pushing by the mother or gentle body traction does not bring the second arm down, attempt to deliver the nuchal arm with pressure along the humerus. If this is unsuccessful, rotate the fetal body by grasping the free arm and bringing it across the chest. By then the second arm should be down or easily reached.

If attempts to deliver the arms fail, it is time to suspect either an unexpectedly large fetus or poor maternal relaxation. Rapid muscle and uterus relaxing anesthesia is needed. This should have been discussed earlier. This is not a time for analgesia but for surgical level anesthesia.

The Aftercoming Head

The major use for the Mauriceau-Snelly-Veight (M-S-V) maneuver is to rotate the aftercoming head into the anteroposterior diameter. The fetal body is still supported, straddled along a supporting arm, and *horizontal* to the floor. In this maneuver some clinicians insert a middle finger into the fetal mouth and place adjacent fingers on the malar eminences to flex the head. Flexion of the fetal head is performed with the M-S-V maneuver. The aftercoming head is more easily flexed by maternal expulsive efforts or by an assistant from the abdominal side. If the head has not delivered spontaneously, now is the time for the assistant to apply suprapubic pressure and flex the head into the pelvis for delivery.

The delivery of the aftercoming head must be controlled so that birth of the head is not rapidly expulsive. A vaginal hand applied in the M-S-V maneuver can control the birth of the head. Rapid birth of the head results in rapid expansion of the compressed fetal bones and may be traumatic to the dural vessels.

At all times during the delivery, the body is kept horizontal to the floor. Quadriplegia may result from hyperextension resulting from elevating the body above the horizontal, or from excessive traction in attempts to flex the aftercoming head through the pelvis. As noted, when a problem exists, flexion is best performed from the abdominal side or with use of Piper forceps.

The Piper Forceps

If spontaneous birth has not occurred, and suprapubic pressure has not succeeded, proceed without delay to use the Piper forceps. The application of these forceps is best described in formal texts. However, a few comments will be made about the procedure.

The blades are applied with the operator kneeling on the floor. If the operator is not low enough, the forceps blades cannot be placed alongside the fetal head. The blades are applied in an upward manner following the sacral curve. If the operator is seated on a stool, the position may be too high. In that higher position, the tendency is to insert the forceps horizontally, which will be obstructed by the sacrum.

The fetus is supported horizontally by an assistant. One forcep is held by the handle, and the tips of the fingers of the second hand should be placed along the end of the forceps blade. In the vagina, the fetal head will still be felt with the fingertips of one hand while guiding the blade inside the cervix (if it is present) with the other hand. A common Piper forceps application error is to insert the blade under the mandible or the jaw of the fetus, thereby blocking insertion of the forceps blade. This is avoided by feeling for the fetal neck and then the jaw with the fingers placed ahead of the forceps blade. In addition, draw the handle of the forceps toward the midline. This moves the forceps blade away from the midline, and the blade can be felt to go around the mandible and along the head of the fetus. The inserted blade is held by an associate, while the operator is still in the kneeling position and the process is repeated. The blades are locked and traction flexes the head under the pubic symphysis.

Head, Neck, and Body Position

Quadriplegia may arise from hyperextending the fetal head, or following the use of excessive traction on the body of the fetus. Whether born by cesarean or vaginal birth, the fetal body must be kept at or below the horizontal plane of the floor. Do not attempt to flex the fetal head by raising the body above the horizontal. The head cannot be flexed in that manner, and doing so can only incur trauma to the fetal neck.

In delivery by cesarean, this principle also must be kept in mind. Don't elevate the body to ease the head out of the incision. The same damage can occur.

Emotions of Vaginal Breech Birth

By the time one reads through the problems surrounding the breech birth, it is not surprising that cesareans have become so common. The physical and emotional stress to the clinician surrounding the breech birth is duplicated nowhere else in obstetrical patient care. Yet, despite this inner disquiet and the struggle to obtain good data, it is suggested that at all birth weights good clinical judgment allows for a vaginal birth route choice.

The key points in the process of a breech birth have been described but this discussion must be considered to be incomplete. The other part of an obstetrician's education is clinical experience, and it should occur at the bedside, hopefully, in the presence of a physician who is comfortable with the breech delivery.

SUMMARY

1. The birth route choice for the frank breech presentation should be arrived at after discussions with the patient and family whenever possible. Chart notes should document all discussions.
2. Between 24 and 36 weeks of gestation radiologic or ultrasonographic evaluation of the fetus should take place if the fetal presentation is breech during two consecutive visits.
3. Ultrasonography is used for fetal morphology. Karyotype studies of the fetus should be performed when indicated.
4. In an environment where emergency care may be given, antepartum cephalic version should be attempted near 37 weeks of gestation.
5. Routine radiographic or sonographic review of head position to confirm flexion, monitoring to confirm absence of fetal distress, and pelvic and fetal size evaluation should take place at the start of labor, with the results written in the patient's chart.
6. The labor may be augmented with oxytocin, but in general the need for responding to abnormalities of labor lowers the threshold for choice of cesarean.
7. Analgesia and anesthesia should be available and used as needed.
8. If possible, a second obstetrician or other support person should be available for the delivery. A pediatrician or support person for the neonate should be present.
9. The clinician is encouraged, if possible, not to intervene during the birth process; neither to pull or extract the fetus.
10. Piper forceps should be available on the delivery table and applied if spontaneous vertex delivery does not take place.

REFERENCES

1. Rosen MG, Chik L: The effect of delivery route on outcome in breech presentation. Am J Obstet Gynecol 1984;148:909–914.
2. Rosen MG, Debanne S, Thompson K, Bilenker R: Long term neurological morbidity in breech and vertex births. Am J Obstet Gynecol 1985;151:718–720.
3. Bodmer B, Benjamin A, McClean FH, Usher PH: Has the use of cesarean section reduced the risks of delivery in the preterm breech presentation? Am J Obstet Gynecol 1986;154:244–250.
4. Morrison JC, Myatt RE, Martin JN Jr, et al: External cephalic version of the breech presentation under tocolysis. Am J Obstet Gynecol 1986;154:900–903.
5. Federle MP, Cohen HA, Rosenwein M, Brant-Zawadzki MN, Conn CE: Pelvimetry NY digital radiography: a low-dose examination. Radiology 1982;143:733–735.
6. James FM III: Anesthetic considerations for breech or twin delivery. Clin Perinatol 1982;77–94.

Chapter 15

Summary
A Philosophy of Labor Management

OVERVIEW

Today the obstetrician practices in a time when cesarean birthrates have been the subject of increasing public scrutiny. Major reasons for the yearly increase in the cesarean birthrate are the increased repeat cesarean, the increased use of the diagnosis of fetal distress, and the increased diagnosis of dystocia. Many patient care problems have been presented in this book to assist the clinician in the art of patient care, and to urge more consistent patterns of management to encourage vaginal birth.

OBJECTIVES

At the conclusion of this chapter, the clinician should:

1. Understand the philosophical elements of obstetrical care during labor and delivery
2. Understand the relationships between obstetrical care and infant neurologic outcome
3. Be able to make clinical decisions and weigh the many patient care choices in an orderly manner
4. Understand the reasons for the rising cesarean birthrate and be able to evaluate the associated patient care decisions in a more critical manner

VAGINAL BIRTH FOLLOWING CESAREAN

Vaginal birth following cesarean is accepted today by most clinicians, but practiced with less than full enthusiasm. Vaginal birth following most primary low transverse cesarean sections should be expected and accepted by the physician and patient. Mothers and family members should receive appropriate education so that the fears of previous labor experiences may be explained and allayed. It is an indication of an obstetrician's attitude and regard for the data if most of his or her previous cesarean patients are not offered and do not pursue a trial of labor in the next gestation. The data published almost monthly in the literature documents the success of this policy and needs no further verification here.

FETAL DISTRESS

The increased use of the diagnosis of fetal distress is difficult to either explain or justify. In the past 15 years no new information has been learned about heart rate monitoring and the diagnosis of fetal distress. The criteria for monitoring findings are unchanged; yet, the diagnosis of fetal distress occurs more frequently. It is evident that the diagnosis is being confused. The many pressures existent at the labor scene move the clinician more rapidly to the cesarean birth route. It would appear that the clinician has moved from a diagnosis of fetal distress because of existing data, to a "question" or a "possibility" of fetal distress. The treatment of this suspicious zone with cesareans is not likely to lead to any reduction in infant morbidity or mortality.

DYSTOCIA

A major portion of this book has been written about the diagnosis of dystocia, which is the basis for a large percentage of primary cesarean births. The use of a language with the same meaning to all is critical. The Friedman nomenclature has withstood the test of time; it is still accurate and allows each clinician to speak in a mutually understood tongue.

With use of the Friedman criteria, given an understanding of what is usual and normal, appropriate treatment programs are available. All too often labors are interrupted without adequate trials. These guidelines will be helpful if used.

However, the use of these labor criteria are only guidelines. Arbitrary termination of labor because the labor deviates from the normal labor curve, or the labor is taking longer than expected, is unacceptable. It is in these situations that the clinician who understands risk and attendant morbidities, and learns to apply judgment rather than to find an excuse for ending the more difficult labors excels. Patience in following a labor and appropriate nonsurgical interventions in the management of labor are the essence of the practice of obstetrics.

Index

A

Abdomen, maternal
  determination of fetal size, lie, position, 38–39
  evaluation at admission, 38–40
  examination complementing vaginal examination, example, 39
  palpation using maneuvers of Leopold, 39–40
Acidosis, association of fetal subarachnoid hemorrhage with, 10
Ambulation
  intervention method
    active phase labor, 103
    latent phase labor, 68
  treatment during latent phase of labor, 74
Amniotic membranes
  artificial rupture
    active intervention in latent phase of labor, 56
    decision of whether or not to rupture, 100
    during latent phase of labor, 58–59
    early intervention, questionable labor, example, 134
    effect on length of labor, 99
    guidelines, 55
    intervention method, failure to make progress after oxytocin, 69
    management problem following, example, 70
    therapeutic choice, nonoccurrence of dilatation, 84
    therapeutic intervention, prolongation, arrest cervical dilatation, 131
    treatment during latent phase of labor, 74
    treatment method for arrested labor, 100
  higher incidence of premature rupture in breech presentation, 174
    and length of labor, 99–100
  rupture
    during latent phase of labor, 53
    and length of latent phase of labor, 55
Analgesia
  intervention method, second stage of labor, 110
  patient management during latent phase of labor, 58
  use during latent phase of labor, 57
Anesthesia. *See also* Epidural anesthesia
  conduction, during latent phase of labor, 59
  intervention method, second stage of labor, 110
  patient management during latent phase of labor, 58
  regional, intervention method for active phase of labor, 103
  use during breech birth, 189
Anteroposterior diameter, 159
Apgar score, and cerebral palsy risk, 16
Arms, nuchal, delivery of in breech birth, 190

Artificial rupture of membranes (AROM). *See* Amniotic membranes, artificial rupture
Asphyxia
association of subarachnoid hemorrhage with, 10
definition of terms, 7
example of poor placental supply confounded by prematurity and labor, 8
neuropathology of brain damage due to, 9–12
perinatal
association with cerebral palsy, 16
brain damage, 7–8
Asynclitism
correction, forceps use for, 162
fetal movement through pelvis, 147
posterior parietal, use of Barton forceps for delivery, example, 168

B

Back, fetal, palpation by maneuver of Leopold, 40
Barton forceps, example of use, 168
Beta hemolytic streptococcus, danger of infection from after membrane rupture, 53
Birth canal problems, labor abnormality, 142
Bleeding. *See also* Hemorrhage
fetal and neonatal, types, 9
intracerebral, in low-birth-weight fetus, 167
intracranial, as endpoint of perinatal asphyxia, 9
Blood loss, following cesarean birth, 3
Blood pressure, elevated, treatment, latent phase of labor, 81
Blood vessels, immature in low-birth-weight fetus and risk of intracerebral hemorrhage, 11
Brain, fetal
association of pathology with function, 13–14
inability to test for damage in utero, 15
intrapartal damage, 15–16
linkage of cerebral pathology with clinical damage, 13
plasticity, 13
Brain damage
asphyxia
neuropathology of, 9–12
pathophysiology, 7–8
categories of pathology, 6
infant, linkage with labor, 6–18
fetal, avoiding, 14–15
Breech birth
aftercoming head in, 191
anesthesia, 189
danger of quadriplegia resulting from hyperextension, 191, 192
emotional problems of, 192
episiotomy, 189–190
extended head, 189
fetal body support during, 190
mechanics, 188–192
need for obstetrical support, 189
neonatal care, 189
nuchal arms, 189, 190
palpation of umbilical cord during, 190
traction during, 190–191
trauma of rapid birth of head, 191
use of Piper forceps, 191–192
Breech presentation, 172–179
already damaged fetus, example, 15
antepartum considerations, 183
appropriateness of vaginal delivery, 180
cesarean delivery in case of high-birth-weight fetus, 174
Cleveland study, neonatal neurologic morbidity and choice of birth route, 176
clinician's decision affected by risk of malpractice accusation, 176
confounding variables, 173–174
decisions regarding during labor, 185
delivery, 180–193
determination by maneuver of Leopold, 40
and different fetal movement, 174
documentation with ultrasonography, 183
evaluation prior to labor, 181–183
fetal anomalies in, 173
fetal umbilical cord sampling in, 183
fetal weight as confounding variable, 177
higher incidence in low-birth-weight infant, 174
higher incidence of in utero infection, 174
higher incidence of premature rupture of membranes, 174
hyperextended vs. flexed fetal head, 187
importance of fetal monitoring during labor, 187–188
intravenous lines used, 188
low-birth-weight fetus, 187
pain medication, 188
percentage delivered by cesarean, 172
performance of external version, example, 181–182
possible abnormal neurologic function, 174
risk variables, 174

term, external version, 183–185
ultrasonography for evaluation, 173
unexpected during labor, example, 185–186
use of oxytocin discouraged, 188
X-ray pelvimetry for, 45
Brow presentation, delivery, 147

C

Caput
correlation with fetal size and labor length, 147
and determination of length of labor, 42
determination by vaginal examination, 42
Caput formation, confounding factor in evaluating vertex descent, 96
Cephalhematomata, incidence of with use of midforceps, 156
Cephalopelvic disproportion, 138–139. *See also* Clinical pelvimetry
diagnosis of during second stage of labor, 108
Cerebral edema
associated with cell necrosis, 12
diagnosed with computerized tomography and ultrasonography, 12
occurrence in term infant, 12
reaction to injury, 12
Cerebral palsy
associated with subdural hemorrhage, 10
category of infant brain damage, 6
effect of fetal maturity at time of brain injury, 14
rates, 3
relationship to labor, 16
Cervical dilatation
arrest of, 91–92
in active phase labor, example, 126–127
after artificial rupture of membranes, 55
average amount of for admission to labor and delivery room, 24
charting during active phase of labor, 88
and determination of length of labor, 41
during accelerative phase of active labor, 88
during decelerative phase of active labor, 91
during maximum dilatation phase of active labor, 91
5 cm as end of latent phase of labor, 64
full dilatation marks beginning of second stage of labor, 107
full dilatation required for forceps application, 163
indicator of active phase of labor, 87
and length of labor, 99
in nullipara vs. multipara, 50–53
maximum rate of, 125–126
median for at time of admission for labor, 50
nonoccurrence, therapeutic choices, 84
and prediction of length of labor, 54
prelabor, example of, 64
primary and secondary arrests, 127–128
protraction, 91–92, 127
and arrest, example, 129–132
range upon admission, 52
rate of in active phase of labor, 124
rate of in decelerative phase of labor, 126–127
relationship to cervical effacement, 101
relationship to vertex descent shown on labor graph, 20–21
requirement for true labor, 48–49
Cervical effacement
and determination of length of labor, 41
effect of artificial rupture of membranes, 102
effect on length of labor, 101
Cervical position, and length of labor, 101
Cervix, vaginal examination, 41–42
Cesarean delivery
birthrates, 1
blood loss following, 3
in case of high-birth-weight breech presentation, 174
choice of during arrest of vertex descent, second stage of labor, 114
Cleveland study, in breech presentation, 176–178
during latent phase of labor, 60, 70–71
emergency
explanation of to patient, 34–35
maternal mortality following, 3
indications for inaccurate during latent phase of labor, 47
infant outcome, comparison with forceps delivery, 156
intervention method
active phase labor, 103
second stage of labor, 105
and low-birth-weight fetus, 167
maternal mortality and morbidity due to, 2–3
need for hospital policy, 48
not easily accomplished at stations +3 and +4, 160
as option with high-birth-weight fetus, 146
percentage of breech presentations delivered by, 172
performance during second stage of labor, 120

Cesarean delivery [*cont.*]
rate of infection following, 3
repeat, and dystochia, 140
treatment
intervention in abnormal active and second stage labor, 118–119
intervention in latent phase of labor, 74
vaginal birth following, 195
Chart documentation, during labor, 20, 27–29
Childbirth education, 23
Cleveland Midforceps Program, 155–156
Clinical examination, upon admission, 37–46
Clinical pelvimetry, 41, 43–45. *See also* Cephalopelvic disproportion; X-ray pelvimetry
effect on length of labor, 101
Cognitive dysfunction, associated with subdural hemorrhage, 10
Computerized tomography
diagnosis of cerebral edema, 12
evaluation of for pelvic measurements, 144, 187
use for breech presentation, 45
Conduction anesthetic, during latent phase of labor, 59
Contractions, uterine
as beginning of latent phase of labor, 48
assessment of force of, 148–150
criteria for effective, 150
insufficient for judging labor, 150
onset defines beginning of latent phase of labor, 6
physiology, 150

D
Delivery, physician presence during, 24–26
Delivery room
environment, 33–35
general conduct in, 22–23
Demerol, treatment, protracted active phase labor, 148
Deprivation of supply, extent of, 10
Descent. *See* Vertex, descent
Diagonal conjugate
length of as problem in labor, 142
measurement of, 44
Dilatation, cervical. *See* Cervical dilatation
Dura mater, lacerations of larger veins and subdural hemorrhage, 9–10
Dystocia, 138–152
abnormal labor, and risk for neurologic injury to fetus, 103
assessment in second stage of labor, 108
criteria for defining, 140–141
diagnosis before end of active phase of labor, 86
diagnosis of with Friedman criteria, 195–196
and fetal brain damage, 139–140
and fetal distress, 136
example, 8
and forceps use, 165
and repeat cesareans, 140
shoulder, 102, 145
treatment program, active management program, 151–152

E
Edema
as endpoint of perinatal asphyxia, 9
cerebral. *See* Cerebral edema
Elective forceps, as unacceptable term, 166. *See also* Forceps
Electronic monitoring. *See* Fetal monitoring
Epidural anesthesia
oxytocin augmentation during second stage of labor, 117
and possible use of forceps, 110
therapeutic intervention, protraction, arrest of cervical dilatation, 131
use of oxytocin after, 110
Epidural block
intervention method, second stage of labor, 110
patient management, latent phase of labor, 58
treatment
during latent phase of labor, 74
protracted active phase labor, 148
Epilepsy
category of infant brain damage, 6
rarely associated with birth process, 16–17
Episiotomy, use of during breech birth, 189–190
Extended head, breech birth, 189
External version, in case of breech presentation, example, 181–182

F
Face presentation
delivery, 146–147
determination by maneuver of Leopold, 40
False labor, 76
management of, 59
no cervical dilatation present, 48
Fetal brain damage, and dystochia, 139–140

Fetal distress
  association with external version of breech presentation, 185
  determination of with fetal scalp blood examination, 136
  during active or second stage labor, 135–136
  explanation of to patient, 34–35
  increased diagnosis of, 195
  indication for forceps intervention, 164–165
Fetal monitoring
  and artificial rupture of membranes, 55
  during active and second stage labor abnormalities, 120
  during administration of oxytocin, 120
  importance during labor in breech presentation, 187
  use during external version of breech presentation, 184–185
Fetal position, abnormality of labor, 142
Fetal presentation, labor abnormality, 142
Fetal scalp blood examination, determination of fetal distress, 136
Fetal size. *See also* High-birth-weight fetus; Low-birth-weight fetus
  evaluation of as problem, 65–66
  excessive, definition, 102
  guideline for forceps use, 163
  labor abnormality, 142
  risk factor in second stage of labor, 109
Fetus
  assessment of abnormalities, 145–146
  assessment of size, 145–146
  avoidance of intrapartum brain damage, 3
  decrease in perinatal mortality rates, 3–4
  determination of size by ultrasonography, 146
  distress and artificial rupture of membranes, 55
  documentation of position by palpation of maternal abdomen, 38–40
  documentation of position by vaginal examination, 40–43
  electronic monitoring, 30. *See also* Fetal monitoring
  evaluation of during latent phase of labor, 65–66
  low-birth-weight group as high-risk population, 4
  mechanics of movement through pelvis, 146–147
  movement different in breech presentation, 174
  risk for replaces maternal risk, 3–4
  size effect on length of labor, 102
  size, lie, and position determined by examination of maternal abdomen, 38–40
Flexion, determination of by vaginal examination, 41–42
Fontanels, position of and estimating flexion and asynclitism, 41
Forceps
  application of and knowledge of ischial spines, 144
  as second stage of labor intervention method, 105
  association of subdural hemorrhage, 10
  caution of use with high-birth-weight fetus, 146
  classification, based on pelvic station and vertex position, 159
  classification by pelvic station and vertex position, 160–161
  clinical indications for, 164–167
  decreased use of with introduction of oxytocin, 155
  elective, as unacceptable term, 166
  failed, 170
  fenestrated, asynclitism, 162
  guidelines for use, 161–164
  historical background and debate, 153–157
  history of use, 106, 154–155
  intervention method
    second stage of labor, 117–118
    of vertex station S+2/S+3, 118
  and low-birth-weight fetus, 166–167
  norms for acceptable traction, 170
  possible use of after epidural anesthesia, 110
  practical considerations, 158–171
  teaching, elective application as unacceptable, 166
  technical considerations for use, 167–170
  traction with, 168–169
    direction and the pelvic curve, 169–170
    and pelvimetry, 144
  trial, 170
  types, 168
  use of in breech birth, 191–192
  use of to shorten second stage of labor, 117
  with overlapping shanks, 168
Forceps delivery, infant outcome, comparison with cesarean birth, 156
Friedman criteria, use in diagnosis of dystochia, 195
Friedman curves, charting of cervical dilatation, 88
Friedman's definitions of labor, 19–20
Fundus
  estimation of height with maneuver of Leopold, 39–40

Fundus [*cont.*]
pressure and vertex descent, 41
pressure of to determine pelvic capacity, 43

G

Group practice, and physician presence during labor and delivery, 26

H

Head
aftercoming, delivery of in breech birth, 191
fetal. *See also* Vertex
determination of engagement by maneuver of Leopold, 40
Hematoma, subdural, fetal, 9–10
Hemorrhage
fetal and neonatal, types, 9
intracerebral, 11–12
categories of, 12
intracranial, in low-birth-weight fetus, 167
postpartum, association with prolonged second stage of labor, 106–107
subarachnoid, 10–11
confounding risk for, example, 10–11
risk factors, 11
subdural
developmental pathology associated with, 10
fetal, 9–10
High forceps, definition, 159
High-birth-weight fetus
and occurrence of shoulder dystocia, 145
breech presentation in, 174
caution
with forceps intervention, 146
with oxytocin intervention, 146
cesarean as option, 146
definition, 102
evaluation of as problem, 65–66
Hospital, patient choice, 31
Hospital environment, importance of, 286
Hydrocephalus, congenital, in breech presentation, 173

I

Infant, brain damage, linkage with labor, 6–18
Infection
after rupture of membranes, 53
rates following cesarean birth, 3
in utero, higher incidence in breech presentation, 174
Intracerebral bleeding. *See* Bleeding, intracerebral
Intracranial bleeding. *See* Bleeding, intracranial
Intrapartum care, breech presentation, 187–188
Ischial spines. *See also* Clinical pelvimetry
and location of molding, 42
estimating prominence of, 44
knowledge of and application of forceps, 144
prominence of as problem in labor, 143

K

Kielland forceps, 168

L

Labor
adequate trial of, 60
arrest
due to insufficient uterine contractions, 148–150
membrane rupture as method of treatment, 100
chart documentation, 20, 27–29
clinical examination, 37–46
decelerative phase, 126
decisions during regarding breech presentation, 185–186
determining length
by cervical dilatation, 54
by pelvic station of vertex, 54
difficult, definitions of, 139
difficulty in determining onset, example, 49
dysfunctional, 150–151
estimation of length by clinical pelvimetry, 43–45
evaluation of forces of, 66
example of no-progress situation, 29
Friedman's definitions, 19–20
guide to care during, 19–36
individualized care, 24
inducement of after rupture of membranes, 53
labor graphs, 20–22
length
and amniotic membranes, 99–100
and cervical dilatation, 99
effect of cervical effacement, 101
effect of cervical position, 101
effect of clinical pelvimetry, 101
effect of fetal size on, 102
effect of patient care environment, 102
effect of vertex position, 101

and pelvic station, 98–99
variables affecting, 100–102
linkage of infant brain damage with, 6–18
long versus short, determination by vaginal examination, 41–43
meaning of numbers defining progress in, 22
measurement of pelvic capacity, 43–45
median dilatation at time of admission, 50
morbidity in management of, 1–5
mortality in management of, 1–5
normal and physician presence, 26
parity and length of, 97
patterned medication use, 24
physician presence during, 24–26
predicting progress by vaginal examination, 40–43
prediction of course of using cervical dilatation rate, 125–126
problem of uncertain onset, 72–76
prolonged, defining, 123
questionable, early intervention, example, 132–235
relationship to
cerebral palsy, 16
epilepsy, 16–17
mental retardation, 16–17
risk during and physician presence, 25
transition from latent to active phase, 124
unsatisfactory progress and artificial rupture of membranes, 55
vaginal examination, 40–43
Labor, abnormal
assessment of fetal abnormalities, 145–146
assessment of fetal size, 145–146
etiologies for, 141–142
and forceps use, 165
inappropriate terms for, 141
measurement of birth canal, 142–144
problem of maternal stature, 142
Labor, active and second stage
abnormalities, example, 118
abnormalities and rate of midforceps use, 156
fetal distress during, 135–136
Labor, active phase, 86–104
abnormalities, therapeutic interventions, 128–135
accelerative phase, 88
arrest of, methods of intervention, 127
assessment of dilatation in, 92–94
cervical dilatation as indicator of, 87
chart notes and analyzation, 128
charting of cervical dilatation during, 88
criteria for, 50–53
decelerative phase, 92
definitions of, 124
early onset, example, 125
factors confounding evaluation of vertex descent, 96–100
interventions, 103
management of abnormalities, 123–137
maximum dilatation phase, 91
protraction of, example, 92–94
slow acceleration, example, 87
three subdivisions, 88
vertex descent phases, 94–96
Labor, latent phase, 47–61
abnormalities and rate of midforceps use, 156
active intervention, 56
example, 81–84
ambulation, method of intervention, 68
analgesia during, 58
artificial rupture of membrane during, 58–59
caput and vertex molding in, 147
cesarean during, 60, 70–71
definition, 48–53, 63–64
diagnosis and treatment, example, 72–76, 78–80
diagnostic routines, 63–71
difficulty in diagnosing onset, example, 67
duration, 52
early intervention, example, 67
end of, 64
epidural anesthesia during, 58
evaluation of carrier, 65
evaluation of passenger, 65–66
factors affecting, 54–55
format for analyzing, 71
indications for cesarean inaccurate during, 47
induction during, example, 50
interval of, 64
management of, 56
following artificial rupture of membranes, example, 70
maternal age and length of, 54
no active intervention, 56–57
onset of, 64
active phase, 50–53
oxytocin augmentation during, 58
oxytocin intervention method, 68–69
parity and length of, 54
patience as method of intervention, 68
patience during, 58
patient better at home, 49
patient position during, 59
rate of cervical dilation in, 63
regional anesthesia during, 58
rupture of amniotic membranes and length of, 55

Labor, latent phase, [*cont.*]
ruptured amniotic membranes during, 53
sedation during, 58
six interventions for patient management, 57–59
subdivisions of, 63
termination because of maternal or fetal distress, 47
therapeutic interventions, 67–71
treatment of abnormalities, 62–85
treatment of lengthy, 70
use of
analgesics, 57
morphine, 57
oxytocin, 57
Labor, second stage, 105–122
abnormal and fetal monitoring, 120–121
abnormalities, 108–109
analgesia as method of intervention, 110
anesthesia as method of intervention, 110
arrest of vertex descent and choice of cesarean, 114
beginning and end of, 105
cesarean as method of intervention, 105
clinical interventions, 109–118
definitions, 107–108
for protracted and arrested, 107
evolution of management, 106
forceps as intervention method, 105
interventions, 105
management of abnormalities, 123–137
normal descent during, 108
oxytocin as method of intervention, 112
patience as method of intervention, example, 110
performance of cesarean during, 120–121
two-hour rule, 106
use of forceps to shorten, 117
vacuum extractor as method of intervention, 105
Labor diagnosis, criteria for, 141
Labor forces, abnormality of labor, 142
Labor graphs, 20–21
Labor management, philosophy of, 194–196
Labor room
crisis in, 1–5
environment, 33–35
evaluation and chart documentation, 27
general conduct in, 22–23
patient choice, 31–33
patient sensitivity, 31–33
progress notes, 28–29
Left occiput anterior rotation, midforceps classification, 159
Leopold, maneuver of, for palpation of maternal abdomen, 39–40
Low forceps, definition, 153, 159, 160
Low midforceps, definition, 159
Low-birth-weight fetus
association of subarachnoid hemorrhages with, 10
breech presentation, 187
vaginal vs. cesarean delivery, 175
and cesarean delivery, 167
high incidence in breech presentation, 174, 175
immaturity of blood vessels and risk of intracerebral hemorrhage, 11–12
increased risk for prolapse of umbilical cord, 174
intracerebral bleeding in, 167
intracranial hemorrhage in, 167
and use of forceps, 166–167

M

Malpractice accusations, effect on treatment choice during labor, 4
Maternal age, and length of latent phase of labor, 54
Maternal exhaustion, use of forceps in second stage of labor, 117–118
Maternal size, as risk factor in second stage of labor, 109
Maternal-fetal disproportion, 65
Maturity, fetal. *See also* low-birth-weight fetus; Prematurity as confounding element in fetal supply risk, example, 8
and intracerebral hemorrhage, 11
and morbidity in breech presentation, 177–178
Mauriceau-Snelly-Wright maneuver, rotation of aftercoming head in breech birth, 191
Meconium
amnioscopy to monitor in latent phase of labor, 82
presence of and artificial rupture of membranes, 55
Medication
as intervention for active phase labor, 103
as treatment during latent phase of labor, 74
Mental retardation
association with birth process, 16–17
category of infant brain damage, 6
Meperidine
therapeutic intervention, protraction and arrest of cervical dilatation, 131
treatment, lengthy latent phase of labor, 70

Midforceps
  data from Cleveland Midforceps Program, 155–156
  definition of terms, 153, 159
  use of and incidence of cephalhematomata, 156
Molding
  and determination of length of labor, 42
  determination by vaginal examination, 42
Morbidity
  fetal, risk during second stage labor, 123
  in management of labor, 1–5
  infant, and breech presentation, 173–174
  maternal, due to cesarean birth, 3
Morphine, treatment
  lengthy latent phase of labor, 70
  possible contraction problem, 66
  use during latent phase of labor, 57
Mortality
  fetal, low-birth-weight group as high risk, 4
  infant, and breech presentation, 173–174
  in management of labor, 1–5
  maternal
    due to cesarean birth, 2–3
    rates, 2
  perinatal, decrease in rates, 3
Mother
  and childbirth education, 22–23
  clinical examination upon admission, 37–46
  evaluation of during latent phase of labor, 65
  maternal stature as problem in labor, 142
Motor dysfunction, associated with subdural hemorrhage, 10
Multipara
  abnormal labor patterns in, 92
  arrested second stage of labor, 107
  criteria for diagnosing
    arrest of descent, 141
    arrest of dilatation, 141
    entry into active phase of labor, 50
    prolonged latent phase, 141
    protracted active phase dilatation, 141
    protracted descent, 141
  failure of vertex descent, treatment, 112
  and length of labor, 97
  and occurrence of uterine rupture with use of oxytocin, 151
  protracted second stage of labor, 107
  protraction
    and arrest of cervical dilatation in, 91
    of cervical dilatation, active phase labor, 127
  rate of cervical dilation in, 63
    in active phase labor, 124
  time of descent, 43
  vertex descent in second stage of labor, 108
  vertex station and length of labor, 99
Muscle relaxants, uterine, use during external version of breech presentation, 184

N

Neurologic function, possibly abnormal in breech presentation, 174
Nuchal arms, breech birth, 189, 190
Nulligravida, length of latent phase of labor, 53
Nullipara
  abnormal labor patterns in, 92
  and length of labor, 97
  arrested second stage of labor, 107
  criteria for diagnosing
    arrest of descent, 141
    arrest of dilatation, 141
    entry into active phase of labor, 50
    prolonged latent phase, 141
    protracted active phase dilatation, 141
    of protracted descent, 141
  pelvic station at beginning of second stage of labor, 108
  protracted second stage of labor, 107
  protraction and arrest of cervical dilatation in, 91
    active phase labor, 127
    example, 129
  rate of cervical dilatation in active phase labor, 124
  vertex station and labor length, 99

O

Oblique vertex position, flow or outlet forceps classification, 159
Obstetrical evaluation, upon admission, 38–43
Occiput anterior vertex birth, 143
Occiput posterior birth, 143
Occiput posterior vertex, low forceps classification, 160
Occiput transverse position, midforceps classification, 160
Outlet forceps, definition, 159, 160
Oxytocin
  active intervention in latent phase of labor, 56
  associated with fetal bradycardia, 120
  augmentation during latent phase of labor, 58
  augmentation with after epidural anesthesia, 117

Oxytocin [*cont.*]
early intervention, questionable labor, 134
failure to make progress following, example, 69
fetal monitoring during administration, 120
induction of labor during possible latent phase of labor, 50
intervention method
active phase labor, 103
latent phase of labor, 68–69
second stage of labor, 112
introduction of use and decreased use of forceps, 155
not associated with fetal brain damage, 140
occurrence of uterine rupture
in multiparous patients, 151
with use in nulliparous patients, 151
therapeutic intervention, arrest, prolongation cervical dilatation, 131
to provide adequate trial of labor, 151
treatment
after epidural anesthesia, 110
arrest of vertex descent, 114
cautioned with high-birth-weight fetus, 146
discouraged in breech presentation, 188
during latent phase of labor, 57
in failure of vertex descent, 112
latent phase of labor, 74, 80, 82
possible contraction problem, 66
protracted active phase labor, 148

P

Pain medication, in breech presentation, 188
Pain relief. See also specific drugs and procedures
demerol, 50
epidural block, example, 24
meperidine, example, 24
morphine, 50
Pajor-Saxtorph maneuver, forceps maneuver, 168
Parity. *See also* Multipara; Nullipara
and length of labor, 97
and length of latent phase of labor, 54
Patience
intervention method
active phase labor, 103
second stage of labor, example, 110
latent phase labor, 68
needed during breech birth, 189
patient management during latent phase of labor, 58
treatment during latent phase of labor, 72
Patient
care, responsibility for, 26
care environment, effect on length of active phase of labor, 102
choice, example of biasing, 32
position, patient management during latent phase of labor, 59
supply of information to and choice, 31–33
Pelvic capacity. *See also* Cephalopelvic disproportion; Clinical pelvimetry
limited in case of breech presentation, 181
tested during second stage of labor, 108
Pelvic curve, and direction of forceps traction, 169–170
Pelvic kidney, presence of and vertex descent, 99
Pelvic sidewalls, measurement of, 44
Pelvic size, measurements useful for forceps application, 163–164
Pelvic station
classification of forceps by, 160–161
confusion in estimating, example, 42
and determination of length of labor, 43
forceps classification based on, 159
guideline for forceps use, 161–162
and prediction of labor length, 98–99
use of centimeter divisions, 97
vertex descent, 97–100
Pelvimetry, x-ray, 45
Pelvis. *See also* Ischial spines; Pubic symphysis
determination of capacity, 41
and forceps traction, 144
measurement of capacity of, 43–45
stations of, 42–43
X-ray pelvimetry, 45
Periventricular leukoencephalomalacia, 11
Physician presence, during labor and delivery, 24–26
Piper forceps, use of in breech birth, 191–192
Placental separation
as indication for forceps application, 165
possibility during external version of breech presentation, 184
Potters syndrome, in breech presentation, 173
Prematurity
association of intracerebral hemorrhage with, 11
and incidence of breech presentation, 174
Primigravida
length of latent phase of labor, 53
slow acceleration during active phase of labor, example, 87

Primipara
rate of cervical dilation in, 63
time of descent, 43
Pubic symphysis
fetus overriding, 99
flexion and descent of vertex beneath, 144
flexion of head under in breech birth, 192
method of directing vertex under with forceps, 169

Q
Quadriplegia, danger of from hyperextension in breech birth, 191, 192

R
Regional block
as method of intervention, second stage of labor, 110
use for nonoccurrence of dilatation, 84
Rh-negative, sensitization, possible occurrence during external version of breech presentation, 184
Right occiput anterior rotation, midforceps classification, 159
Ritodrine, use during external version of breech presentation, 184
Rotations, and forceps classifications, 159–160

S
Sacrosciatic notch, estimating size, 44
Sacrum
as guideline for forceps use, 162
curve of, estimating, 44
Seconal, treatment, lengthy latent stage of labor, 70
Sedation, as patient management during latent phase of labor, 58
Shoulder dystocia
more common with large sized infants, 102
unpredictability, 145
Simpson-type forceps, 168
Subarachnoid hemorrhage. *See* Hemorrhage, subarachnoid
Subdural hematoma. *See* Hematoma, subdural
Subdural hemorrhage. *See* Hemorrhage, subdural
Support person, in labor room, 22–23
Symphysis pubis. *See* Pubic symphysis

T
Teaching forceps, elective application as unacceptable, 166
Terbutaline, use during external version of breech presentation, 184
Two-hour rule
arrest of vertex descent, 114, 117
second stage of labor, 106

U
Ultrasonography
determination of fetal size, 146
diagnosis of cerebral edema, 12
to document breech presentation, 183
method of estimating fetal size, 66
at start of labor in breech presentation, 187
Umbilical cord
compression, as indication for forceps application, example, 164–165
fetal blood sampling in case of breech presentation, 183
palpation during breech birth, 190
problems during external version of breech presentation, 184
prolapse of after rupture of membranes, 53
prolonged compression, neurologic consequences, 9
risk of prolapse increased in low-birth-weight infant, 174
Uterus. *See also* Contractions, uterine
assessment of force of contractions, 148–150
size, and artificial rupture of membranes, 55

V
Vacuum extractor
indications for use, 170–171
method of intervention, second stage of labor, 105, 117–118
protraction of active phase of labor, 94
use during arrest of vertex descent, 96
versus use of Barton forceps, 168
Vaginal birth, following cesarean, 195
Vaginal dilatation, visualized during labor, example, 39
Vaginal examination
assessment of cervical dilatation during active phase of labor, 92
labor, 40–43
Version, external, breech presentation
example, 181–182
risks, 184

Version, external, breech presentation [*cont.*]
  techniques, 184–185
  term, 183–185
  use of fetal monitoring during for breech presentation, 184–185
  use of uterine muscle relaxants, 184
Vertex
  asynclitism, effect on length of labor, 101
  birth, controlled, with forceps, 170
  descent, arrest and two-hour rule, 114, 117
    arrest, 96, 127
      and forceps use, 165
      oxytocin treatment, 114
    character of normal during second stage labor, 108
    during active phases of labor, 94–96
    failure, use of oxytocin, example, 112
    and fundal pressure, 41
    rate of in active and second stage labor, 127
    relationship to cervical dilatation shown in labor graph, 20–21
  extended, delivery, 146
  flexion of, 144
    correction, forceps use, 162
  molding of, 147–148
  pelvic stations of, 97–100
    and determining length of labor, 54
  position, and determination of length of labor, 41
  sutures of, position of and estimation of flexion, 42
  time of occurrence in primipara and multipara, 43
  vaginal examination, 41–42
Vertex left occiput transverse, asynclitic, 147
Vertex molding
  confounding factor in evaluating vertex descent, 96
  correlation with fetal size and labor length, 147
  degree of as guideline for forceps use, 163
Vertex occiput posterior position, maternal exhaustion and use of forceps, 117
Vertex position
  classification of forceps by, 160–161
  determination with maneuver of Leopold, 40
  effect on length of labor, 101
  forceps classification based on, 159
  must be known for forceps application, 163
Vertex presentation, rotation, descent, and flexion, 146–147
Vertex station S+2/S+3, therapeutic intervention at, 118

X

X-ray pelvimetry, 45
  importance of, 186–187